FITNESS IS A WAR

To Dominate the 30

Endomorph @ War ™
Entry Level Program and Journal

"What You Should Know and WHO You Must Become to <u>Win YOUR War</u> against <u>YOUR</u> Genetics"

Héctor R. Morales- Negrón, PhD,

Certified Mental Performance Consultant (CMPC)

ACSM – Certified Personal Training

U.S. Army Master Fitness Trainer

Founder, PMG: Optimal Performance Education, LLC

Former Director of Personal Fitness at U.S. Military Academy, West Point

FOR SOME: FITNESS IS A WAR TO DOMINATE THE 30

Endomorph @ War ™

Entry Level Program and Journal

"What You Should Know and What You Must Become to Win YOUR War against YOUR Genetics"

Published by Peak Mental Game: Optimal Performance Education, LLC

Printed and distributed by Createspace

7921 112th Avenue East, Parrish, FL 34219

Héctor R. Morales- Negrónpeakmentalgame@gmail.com

850-459-1498

All rights reserved. Except for brief excerpts for review purposes, no part of this book may be reproduced or used in any form without the written permission of the publisher.

ISBN-13: 978-0-9983547-2-9

© 2020 Héctor R. Morales- Negrón. All rights reserved.

Printed in the United States of America

First Edition 2020

TABLE OF CONTENTS

Foreword by *(Find a recognized big person that has been successful and has won many battles)*

Dedication

Acknowledgments

The Author's Personal Battle: Who Am I? Why does this matter to me?

Section One: Welcome to the Battleground - Understanding the Endomorph Challenges to the Head, Heart, and Body

Section Two: The Mental Performance Solution – Who You Must Become

Section Three: Why is it a War? - Planning the War: Assessments, Goal Setting, and Commitment

Section Four: Fitness Foundations through the Endomorph's Eyes - Endomorph Soldier's Rules of Engagement

Section Five: Endomorphs and Nutrition – Basic Rules

Section Six: Endomorph @ War Rules of Engagement for Fitness and Nutrition – Dominate the 30

Section Seven: Joining the E@W Army Community

E@W Level One Program 12-Week Journal

About the Author

Overview

I want to share with you a powerful story. Growing up in Puerto Rico, I embarked on a lifelong journey to redefine success in the fitness and wellness world. From a young age, I fell in love with sports and physical education, despite not having a body type that matched the 'ideal' mold. This inner conflict, combined with the physical challenges I faced, fueled countless sleepless nights, moments of low self-esteem, and frustration. Yet, these struggles also ignited my drive to pursue a fitness journey filled with highs and lows, ultimately leading me to become an Army Master Fitness Trainer and later, the Director of Personal Fitness Development at the United States Military Academy at West Point. There, I helped thousands of soldiers and cadets reach their peak performance.

Through this journey, I learned to embrace who I am. I developed the resilience to push past societal labels that often brand endomorphs as lazy or undisciplined. I also learned what it truly takes to succeed in a competitive world. This program is rooted in those lessons, combining conflict resolution strategies and modified military tactics to help you create a winning plan — against genetics, societal pressure, and, most importantly, the toughest opponent you'll face; yourself.

I invite you to join me and become a soldier in the Endomorph @ War community. Together, we can not only overcome personal battles but also challenge a society that still tolerates discrimination and harassment against those who don't fit the "ideal" body image, regardless of their performance.

Take a moment to reflect. If you answer "yes" to any of these questions, you may be ready for your own battle:

- *Do you struggle to lose weight more than those around you?*

- *Have you been labeled obese by the BMI scale for as long as you can remember?*

- *Can you recall the last time you were within the "suggested" weight or BMI range?*

- *Have you started a fitness program, only to quit because the progress didn't meet your expectations?*

- *Have you succeeded in a fitness program, only to fall back to your starting point due to time constraints or injuries?*

If any of these resonate with you, prepare to shift your mindset. Through this program, you will go from feeling frustrated by your fitness struggles to becoming an Endomorph @ War. You'll gain a deeper understanding of your body, identify what has been holding you back, and arm yourself for a new battle — one fought with the support of a community that stands against the last acceptable form of discrimination in America: body composition and appearance.

Let me be transparent: this program is not about achieving perfection. It's about the fight. I've had moments where I was at my best, and other times when I lost ground. That's the reality of war — armies gain ground and lose it, only to fight harder to win it back. Every endomorph understands this battle. Many have given up — but not you. You're here because you're not done yet. You're ready to join the Endomorph @ War community and fight alongside me. I promise you the real me — the coach, the Army

Master Fitness Trainer, the National Championship Coach, the endomorph who knows your struggle firsthand.

This community isn't for the casual weekend warrior or the person who claims miraculous transformations. This program draws on 30 years of education and experience. I'm here to help you win your battles, one day at a time, with your commitment.

Why did I build this community? Simple—I am an endomorph, period. Growing up, I was always one of the biggest kids. Despite eating the same things as my friends and participating in the same activities, I struggled. It was frustrating. Over the years, I have sought answers, and now that I've found some, I want to share them with you. I want to help you set realistic goals and manage your challenges. This isn't just for adults, but for kids who are growing up in a world where fast food is abundant and physical activity is declining. We must educate ourselves and the next generation about these battles.

After years of study and experience in physical education and exercise science, and with a record of achievement in competitive settings, I know that I'm not lazy or undisciplined. I've accomplished many things, but one thing has still been elusive: keeping the body weight the Army, society, and even my own expectations demanded. I've reached that weight temporarily, but I always returned to my natural state. Therefore, it cannot be about weight, it must be about performance.

There are many theories about why some people gain weight more easily or struggle with hunger. We'll explore those theories together in the upcoming sessions and workshops to help you understand your own battlefield. <u>This program isn't about excuses — it's a strategy guide for your personal war</u>. You must understand your enemy to defeat it, and you must stay engaged in this lifelong fight for a better quality of life. You will become a soldier with a mission, and by staying on the course, you'll know you've done your best to become the best version of yourself. This community is for those in the real struggle. Welcome!

"ACCEPT WHO YOU ARE,

KNOW WHO YOU ARE,

BELIEVE IN WHO YOU CAN BE."

Michelle A. Homme

Dedication

To my kids: Meagan, Hector, and Francisco. They have always driven me to do better and to continue my fight. My daughter is extremely talented and, as an English literature major, has been very instrumental in the completion of this book. Meg, I am very appreciative of all your help and extremely proud of you. My boys are bright and talented in their own pursuits as well and I am also very proud of them. However, I have given these boys something I did not want to hand over. They are endomorphs, just like me. While most of their friends get to look at their family tree, they get to look at their family forest. Because I know the roller coaster of frustrations that I have been on, I want to arm and prepare them for their journey. I gave them a problem and with this approach, I want to give them a solution or at least a path for them to win their genetics battles while at the same time, help you, the reader, embark on your own journey.

To my wife, she met me when I was "skinny" and has seen firsthand what is like to be an endomorph in a competitive environment. She provided me with hugs, encouragement, and learned as much as she could about what it was to be me. Best of all, after more than three decades, she is still here.

Lastly, this book is dedicated to all those professional soldiers I met throughout my military career that could no longer stand the pressure of getting their body measured by, at times, soldiers with lower levels of performance, both professionally and physically. These soldiers live in my memory in the image of Staff Sergeant (SSG) T. As a second lieutenant, on my first assignment as an officer, SSG T was the first soldier I lost to the weight battle. He was one of the best non-commissioned officers I ever served with. He was a great leader and greatly respected by his soldiers. The soldiers under his leadership excelled and he personally did superbly in his physical fitness testing scores; however, he was an endomorph. He probably did not know it, but he was one. SSG T had a hard time maintaining the weight listed on the official tables; because of it, he was always body taped and mocked by some of his peers, even those not in leadership positions. I tried to keep him in, but he was tired. I am certain that he is not the only good leader that had to leave the service because of these personal challenges;

clearly opening doors for the progression and promotion of genetically gifted but not necessarily better soldiers nor leaders. I am sure that these genetically disadvantaged leaders that had to leave still utilized their talents in many areas; but for those that are still in, who go through the same decision making, this book may help you.

Acknowledgements

My gratitude and most sincere appreciation go to Ms. Meagan Camero, who gave from her personal time to provide me with a second set of eyes and help me edit this book.

Lastly, my Judo Daughter **Heather Schuck** for her professional and always available talents as writer. She has been a second set of eyes for many of my manuscripts and for this book. Thank you for being part of this journey.

Introduction:

Author's Personal Battle: Who Am I? Why does this matter to me?

I have always been a happy camper. I think it is part of my personality, so this book is not about complaining or settling any back-burner issues. My family, friends, colleagues, and even subordinates who served with me can confirm sightings of a comedic and energetic Hector that can bring a smile to any audience. I believe that most endomorphs are that way, at least to the outside world. On the inside, however, their self-talk could kill them with the echo of the same criticism they hear from society, their peers, and even their family.

In the next couple of pages, I want to give you a glance at the life and experiences that shaped this author. *As you will find out, "these challenges were met head-on with a performance-driven mindset, where mastering the process, outworking everyone, and consistently achieving the best possible results became a way of life."* As you read, you may feel connected with some of my experiences. If so, I urge you to eventually share those with the Endomorph @ War Army. Let others know that they are not alone in this battle and that there is strength within us.

The Early Years

I was born in Puerto Rico and grew up in the town of Manati. During the 1970s, Manati was a very sports-oriented town where many professional baseball players and other elite athletes originated. My Dad was the town's Sports Director from 1976 until 1980. Thus, from age 9 until I was 13, I accompanied my father to many sports venues and activities throughout the island each weekend. Inevitably, I fell in love with sports, fitness, and competition.

Because of these experiences, I wanted to be around sports and to compete. I remember carrying the Pan American Games torch through the streets of our town for about a mile in 1979. The athletic experience was something I needed to be part of. However, I had a significant challenge; I was a big kid for my age. As a matter of fact, for as long as I can remember, I have always been bigger than my peers. I did not know why nor cared at the earlier stages of my life.

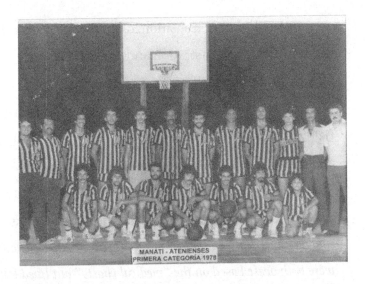

(This is one of many teams my Dad helped develop during those four years. That kid with squeezable cheeks in the bottom right corner is me!)

I became frustrated with some of my peers for not respecting what I was able to do, or appreciating who I was, but nevertheless that was my life. All I wanted to do during that time was play and be part of the experience. As I grew older, I asked myself at times, *why was I different? Why was I bigger than my peers if we practically ate the same school-provided meals) and we did the same sports?* The answers to these questions came much later in my life as I learned to cope with these challenges.

As my father transitioned out of the sports office in 1980, my frustration and curiosity were already at their peak. I remember deciding that physical education and exercise science would be my field of study. I wanted to play and coach, but most of all, I wanted to know what was different about me. There were some things that were obvious - both of my parents were also a bit bigger than the average folks. *(my dad died at 81 and my mom turned 80 in 2024). They were both obese based on the "medical charts" but lived long and active lives.)* I also enjoyed eating - but who doesn't? While I truly enjoyed eating, my friend who was significantly skinnier than me enjoyed eating even more. I am pretty sure we know someone that can eat the way he did. I remember him eating 20 slices of pizza with ease on one occasion. At times, he ate much more but remains thin until this day. These facts always puzzled me, and I always wished that I knew then what I know now.

As the middle school years went by, I saw my weight increase and most of my peers decrease as we started to develop and grow. Not being able to reach your fitness goals takes a toll. It takes an emotional toll that builds a cognitive schema of what you are that is very hard to overcome. Some of these moments of failure empower your inner negative voice and, if this negative self-talk started when you were a kid, that voice will be there until the day you die unless you learn to subdue and overcome it.

One event that shaped my own mental schema happened during the second semester of eighth grade. In our town's high school, they had a military program that we could start as incoming freshmen. The initial phase was a physical test that included pushups, sit-ups and a short run. The pushups station was the first one we encountered, and this station was led by one of my "friends". He did not count one of my pushups. He wrote a zero on my sheet and humiliated me in front of all the other participants. I never completed that test. Immediately after the pushup incident, I left and went home. I can relive this incident in my head as it happened yesterday. I cannot imagine what would have happened if this incident had occurred in today's environment with all the technology, social networking, and messaging capabilities. I would have had to fight my way in and out of school for at least a week!

After that day, something had to change. I could not take it anymore and to make matters worse, the environment in our town was changing. There were fights in high school every day and many of my friends became members of different gangs in the town. My lack of physical fitness, the potential of being a target, and the town changes were a bad combination for a young, out-of-shape freshman about to enter high school; action was needed.

Introduction into the Martial Arts and High School Years

The summer before our high school freshmen year, one of my best childhood friends had the idea to start a group of our own. It was not a gang; for me it had a bigger purpose. We would train in different martial arts to include striking and grappling and we would stick together against other gangs in the town if the need arose. We were members of the Full Contact Squad. We researched martial arts books and learned about fighting strategies. We trained every day with made-up fitness tools such as cement-filled cans for dumbbells and sandbags for weights, many pushups and sit-ups, and fighting training. At times, we would train up to three hours per day. After this engagement with the martial arts, I started to see the first benefits of physical activity in my body. The first day of high school was a different experience for me. Everyone was now amazed at how much more in shape I was compared to what I looked like before we broke for the summer. This experience felt different as I saw others now being the butt of jokes and harassment. I wish I could have done more to help them.

Throughout my high school experience, if I was doing martial arts training, I would be in good shape. If I had an injury or had to work and could not train, the pounds accumulated quickly, and this frustrated me. To stay physically active, I continued to play basketball for hours each day and did martial arts training for the three years of high school, only stopping when I was injured. Every time I stopped; it was back to my body's normal weight. Back then, my go-to weight was between 205 and 210 pounds. At 5'10", that is much more than the desired weight on any table or BMI calculation. However, my body wanted to go there naturally. After our martial arts training group broke up, I continued to focus on combat sports training and remember going with my training buddies to practice Taekwondo, wrestling, and Judo at the beach in our town. While I continued to play basketball, volleyball, and baseball for fun, these three combat sports were the ones that I ultimately stuck with and competed in throughout college and beyond.

College Years

My best childhood friend and I entered the University of Puerto Rico in the Fall immediately after high school graduation. While my childhood experiences had impacted my self-image and self-esteem, shifting my focus from appearance to performance, I had taken control of my self-esteem, confidence, and ability to compete in everything I did. My body still reacted the same and gained weight quicker than most, but I still did not know why. There was no answer to why I gained more weight or why I gained it more easily than those around me with similar habits.

After two years of college, needing additional funding for expenses, my buddy and I entered the U.S. Army as enlisted infantrymen. Neither of us could speak English so we went to a military language school. For the second time in my life, my body's reactions to physical training became clear. Before departing for the military, I told my Judo coach that I would return for my scholarship, and that I would compete in the 189 pounds category. While staying at 189, almost 20 below the mark my body wanted to be, was not going to be an easy task, I made it my purpose to get as fit as I could and to get the best out of the Army experience.

I fully bought into the Army motto of the time, "*Be All You Can Be*". I spent six months in the language school and did physical training (PT) three times a day. The mandatory PT in the morning, immediately after lunch, and 100 pushups and sit-ups at lights out. I was eating more than I ever ate before and yet was getting stronger and getting leaner. After my basic training experience, my physical condition started affecting my psychological traits as well. I was showing a level of confidence and self-esteem that was never noticed before. I received the award for the best physical test scores at Fort Benning, GA and began wearing a patch that stated, "Physical Fitness Excellence". The formerly "out of shape" kid from a small town in Puerto Rico that could not get a single push up counted had the best physical performance of his class. An unbelievable tale, right? My bodyweight was now 192 and performance in all components of fitness had moved from health and wellness to a highly competitive level. I felt confident and ready to take on the world.

After my initial military experience, I returned to the UPR, Judo, and Wrestling team, and joined the ROTC program where my levels of physical fitness gave me an advantage. I conducted physical training sessions for those who were struggling in their physical development and stayed on top of my physical and academic performance. My life was moving in the right direction. I became a National Collegiate Champion and started to show promise to compete at the international level. I forgot about my struggles with weight and appearance. In this world, no one knew the out-of-shape kid and because of my continued level of activity (I was burning over 8,000 calories a day!), competition preparation, and the need of the sport to stay under 189 pounds, my problems with weight seemed to be a problem of the past.

But I was wrong, very wrong.

During my last year in college, injury showed its ugly face yet again. I had not been injured since high school and here I was again, unable to do high calorie-spending physical activity and even when modifying my eating patterns, the weight started to creep back in. In less than two months, I was back above 210 and had to, for the first time, experience the Army's body measurement assessment, called the tape test. When my supervisor conducted the test, I was still achieving perfect physical performance scores; however, he approached me like there was something wrong with me. It was probably the same attitude that two years later drove SSG T to leave the service. The attitude of one individual towards my body composition tape test brought back painful memories. I could have declined my active-duty commission but if you have been following the story closely, you should know by now that this is not my style. I would not give a single person the satisfaction of driving me away. If nothing else, I would use their voice and attitude as a motivator to drive me forward. I was going to accept the challenge. I mean, WE were going to accept the challenge. By graduation time, I had married Marisol, the sister of one of my ROTC peers, and she and I were ready to enter this experience together.

Military Career

In August 1990, Marisol and I reported to Fort Bliss, Texas for the Officer Basic Course. By the time that we arrived, my injury was completely healed, and I was back performing well. I was able to qualify for very physically demanding training obtaining one of the limited slots for Airborne and Air Assault schools and completing both courses with high honors. Our first duty assignment was Fort Polk, Louisiana. The Division was very demanding in terms of hours of work, but I was able to work with great soldiers, including SSG T.

Two new challenges to my genetics started to arise. First, because of the work hours and family schedule my workouts were now limited to the unit physical training sessions in the morning. Second, that to-go weight that used to be 205-210 had now moved up to 215-220. Regardless of what I did, it always went back to that new number. Because of this, I was "taped tested" again several times by subordinate soldiers. The tape test requires a soldier to remove his shirt and have circumferences around the waist and neck taken. I have always believed this to be degrading, especially when I was still wearing the physical fitness excellence patch because of my physical performance.

During my first year at Fort Polk, there were no martial arts training opportunities available in our base other than Taekwondo twice a week. I did Taekwondo, but it was not enough. I needed to return to competition. That was the only way I knew that helped me keep my weight down. In 1992, one single event changed my approach; I needed to get back on the mat.

In the summer of 1992, the Olympics were in Barcelona, Spain. Since the time I carried the Pan American Flame in 1979 when it went through our town, I wanted to be part of these games. I loved to see the athletes' pride in representing their country. That summer, I was watching the opening ceremonies and saw one of my teammates from the University of

Puerto Rico carrying our flag. My heart was filled with joy and pride. This moment motivated me to continue to pursue my Judo journey. I had given up on this journey two years prior when my injury made me change my path. Seeing my friend at the Olympics helped me reconnect with my why and how much I valued the competitive experience.

I found a place an hour away from the base to train twice a week and would travel three hours one way on Saturdays for higher competition training in Houston. I was back on the path and set my sights on my first competition and the return to 189 pounds. With the support of my family, I was able to manage my time and training and return to the 189 for competition. My wife became my day-to-day motivator as she traveled with me to training and competitions. Without her support, nothing would have been possible. Returning to the competition weight was more difficult than before but I always managed to make the scale the day of the competition. Today, because of what I have learned, I question my approach to making weight because I placed myself at risk of injury and limited recovery but those were the strategies of the time.

After 2 years of competitions, I had done well enough to qualify for the Armed Forces Judo camp that would select the team that would represent the U.S. at the First World Military Games. In 1995, I won my division at the Armed Forces Championships and represented the U.S. at the games in Rome. It was a great experience and everything I had dreamed of about international competition and was even selected by my peers to carry the USA Flag for the opening ceremony. I continued training and competition during my tours of service in Germany and Korea, allowing me to stay on top of my weight management. After commanding two units in Germany, Bosnia, Croatia, and Hungary, I was selected as a faculty member in the Department of Physical Education at West Point.

At the academy, I was able to transition from performance to instruction of fitness and wellness and began to fully understand the science behind my challenges. I was also able to start my coaching experience in Judo that has led me to coach U.S. teams to several collegiate and military world championships.

West Point Years

I arrived at the United States Military Academy at West Point for my second tour, this time as an Academy Professor of Physical Education in 2008. In 2010, my boss in the Department of Physical Education gave me the task of leading the personal fitness course for the entire Corps of Cadets. By education and experience, I was extremely qualified for this job. During my military career, I led my platoons, batteries, and sections to the highest physical test scores and to great levels of physical performance in their jobs. I had developed national collegiate Judo champions, had lead group exercise classes to help people improve their physical conditioning and performance, and as a master fitness trainer had helped thousands of soldiers improve their physical performance.

Despite all of this, during the first meeting a civilian professor stated to me "*I don't understand the choice here, they obviously don't care about body composition*", he was referring to me as a choice for the personal fitness director position because I was bigger than all other members of the department. At this time, it was clear that for some people in that environment, how you look is more important than what you can do. This "professor" had never led anyone to anything, and his experience was outside the kinesiology and exercise science field. Nevertheless, my selection was still openly questioned solely on his perception of who should lead this course. Individuals with limited emotional intelligence will always be present; use them as motivation, I have always said.

I know that these situations are not unique to me; they happen in society as well and I am sure that many of you have gone through similar experiences. It is obvious that in our society, most of the fitness "experts" are genetically blessed and don't have the struggles an endomorph individual has. Somehow, they expect us to stay outside "their area" if we do not look like they do. As you can already see, I do not believe that fitness should be exclusive. I will battle through anyone's irrational expectations and lack of emotional intelligence. Obviously, my boss at the Academy was a great man and could see what was important. I led this course for four years before retiring, impacting the lives of thousands of future officers. At the end of the day, impacting others is what matters most, that is why I choose to fight, and that is why I hope you will join me on this journey.

Why Am I Sharing This with You?

I am an endomorph...period! I was always one of the biggest kids in the class; For some reason, food affected me differently than it did my friends. As stated in the story, we were a tight group of friends and ate pretty much the same things. We played the same games and conducted many activities together and yet I was always the one that struggled. It was frustrating and I had to learn more about it. Now that I have learned, I want to share the knowledge with you because it has made my goal setting easier to manage and personal situations easier to handle. I not only want to share with the adults but also with the kids, the ones that are developing now. They have it worse than we had it. Fast food is in abundance and entertainment activities are no longer physical. Even if they were not born endomorphs, once their body changes and creates more fat cells, their bodies will react like one. Being big is still an accepted target for everyone to criticize and opine. We need to educate ourselves and our kids about these battles.

Again, I am an endomorph. After many years in physical education and exercise science searching for an answer, I have come to grips with this reality. I am not lazy or undisciplined. I have accomplished many things in my life; however, there is one thing I have not been able to accomplish: Be at the bodyweight the Army, society, and, at times, my unrealistic expectations wanted me to be. Sure, sometimes, I would make it there - temporarily, with lots of sacrifices, but would always return to my normal state.

There are many theories out there that address why some people gain weight faster than others and why they feel hungry all the time, we will address all these theories in the upcoming chapters and in the courses throughout the community platform to help you better understand your battlefield. Nevertheless, in the eyes of the genetically blessed, we are always at fault, and something is missing in our psychological makeup. You probably have heard it many times: *Just eat less! Make better choices! You don't do it because you don't want to,* etc.

From this story, we took several lessons and integrated them into our **Endomorph @ War** ™ approach but these three are critical for you to keep in mind. First, it does not matter if you were born an endomorph, you can accomplish whatever you want if your goals are performance-based. Second, if you are an endomorph, it is extremely hard work to maintain unrealistic societal expectations. You need to identify what is realistic for you and fight like hell to stay there. Lastly, as soon as you stop being intentional or something gets in the way, genetics will win. Therefore, you must have a plan for when these situations happen. Adaptability is going to be critical.

I have compiled facts in this book to help you understand that there are reasons why you struggle with weight. It is paramount that you understand how these things impact who you are. ***It is not a book to give you excuses; it is a map of your battlefield.*** You need to understand your enemy to defeat it and to stay engaged in this lifelong battle for a better quality of life. You must become a soldier with a specific and realistic mission and by staying on the course, you will never feel like you have not done your very best to be the best version of you that you can be.

Section One: Welcome to the Battleground - Understanding the Endomorph Challenges to the Head, Heart, and Body

"The problem is not the problem. The problem is your attitude towards the problem."- Theodore Isaac Rubin

Introducing the Problem

In today's society, fitness is a universally understood concept but often embraced by only a few. Let's be honest—if fitness could be achieved by a pill, most of us would gladly take it. If wishful thinking alone could transform our bodies, we'd all be in top shape. But reality paints a different picture.

In any given town, about 15% of people are committed to fitness no matter what. Their motivation is deeply rooted in something vital, and they follow a routine that ensures they stay on track. Many in this group are athletes or work in the fitness industry, and they've already found their rhythm. This book isn't for them.

At the opposite end, there's another 15%—those who, despite knowing better, won't change their habits. They might even recognize they're making poor choices, but without a life-or-death ultimatum, they're unlikely to act. Unfortunately, by the time a wake-up call arrives, it's often too late. This book isn't for them either.

You, however, belong to the remaining 70% — people who want to be more active but face barriers. These barriers might include a lack of time, motivation, or frustration from not seeing results despite trying. Within this group are endomorphs, individuals whose body type makes fitness more challenging. You've probably been motivated to start a fitness plan, only to feel discouraged when the results didn't come as expected. Maybe your friend achieved their goal in 90 days, but you didn't. Or worse, you did hit your target, but soon after, you found yourself back at square one. These struggles are why you've picked up this book — to understand why it's harder for you and to find a solution.

This is your turning point, your chance to approach fitness with a new mindset. It's the beginning of your journey from frustration to becoming a warrior — a warrior who understands why your path to fitness is more difficult, and why that's not a weakness.

By the end, you'll know what you're truly up against and be ready to rise to the challenge, integrating fitness into your life as a core part of who you are.

We'll achieve this by tackling a missing link in fitness: education. Too often, fitness "experts" are trained in weekend seminars, with just enough knowledge to tell you what to do but not why. You've likely heard them shout generic advice like "GOOD FORM!" or "YOU'RE HITTING THE WALL!" after a mere 20 minutes. But true fitness goes deeper, especially for those who don't fit the standard mold.

High school physical education has been reduced to an hour a week in many districts, and recreational activities are often replaced by digital distractions. Meanwhile, government attempts to fix the issue focus on cafeteria menus, while ignoring the need for more physical activity. This cookie-cutter approach to fitness leaves those with endomorphic body types at a disadvantage. And if you're an endomorph, chances are your children will face similar challenges in a system not built for them.

This book won't solve the nation's fitness education problem, but it will empower you to understand and overcome the challenges unique to endomorphs. Along the way, you'll learn how to help others, including your children, succeed where the current system fails. Together, we can break the cycle and create a healthier future for ourselves and the next generation.

What is an endomorph?

The endomorph body type is one of the three somatotypes introduced by American psychologist William Sheldon in the 1940s. Sheldon developed this theory to link body types with personality traits, and over time, his model has been used to explore not only these associations but also how society views different body types and their connection to physical activity and fitness development. It's important to recognize that while some may dismiss the relevance of somatotypes in fitness, the challenges faced by individuals at the extremes — endomorphs and ectomorphs — are clear.

Ectomorphs, for example, are typically thin, with a natural tendency to struggle in building muscle or storing fat. In fitness, they often seek out mass gainers and protein supplements, hoping to increase weight and muscle size. On the opposite end of the spectrum are endomorphs, who tend to store fat more easily and may struggle with weight management. In between, mesomorphs—those with naturally muscular builds—enjoy an advantage. They can develop muscle quickly, maintain a low body fat percentage, and often represent the ideal physique many aspire to achieve.

However, it's important to understand that body type is largely determined by genetics, and while you can optimize your fitness, you can't entirely change your somatotype. If you're born with the characteristics of an endomorph, striving to become a mesomorph isn't realistic. Instead, the goal should be to become the best version of yourself—focusing on maximizing your fitness potential within your genetic framework. As the saying goes, if you're born an apple, don't try to be a pear—just be the best apple you can be.

If you're an endomorph, you're probably familiar with how this body type is often characterized: larger bone structure, a wider waist, and a tendency to gain weight quickly. As comedian Sinbad once joked, "You look at a cookie and gain two pounds." Unfortunately, this rings true for many endomorphs, who are predisposed to store fat more easily due to having a higher number of fat cells. Think of it like having a bigger garage — if you have more storage space (fat cells), excess energy that isn't burned off will be stored there.

Interestingly, fat cells aren't just passive storage units; they're active living organisms. This means the number of fat cells you have can influence your hunger levels, as they send signals to your brain regarding energy storage. The average person has around 30 billion fat cells, and as they store energy, they expand. While the number of fat cells you're born with is predetermined, your body can create more if necessary.

Understanding your body type and its tendencies is key to developing a successful fitness strategy. By knowing your "battlefield" and recognizing how your body stores fat, you can craft a plan to manage it effectively and achieve your fitness goals.

What are the most frustrating elements of being an endomorph?

There is a laundry list of things that are frustrating about being an endomorph. The most problematic of all is that people in our society believe that they have the right to opine, and judge based on weight and body composition. For some reason, we have made it acceptable that if a person is bigger, it is okay to poke fun, disrespect, or believe that we know the content of their character. In psychological studies, people of all ages are often shown silhouettes representing the three somatotypes. Endomorphs are frequently labeled as fatter, shorter, older, more old-fashioned, lazier, less physically strong, less attractive, more talkative, and more dependent. If you have an endomorphic body, you face these judgments immediately. The deck is stacked against you socially, and it's crucial to address these perceptions head-on. Your mindset and attitude will play a significant role in overcoming these challenges. For me, going against the norm and outworking everyone became a way of life.

The Bad and How to Fix It

One challenge endomorphs face is the perception of laziness or low energy. As an endomorph, I can admit that I sometimes must fight with myself to get my workouts done. But looking at everything I've accomplished, I can confidently say I am not lazy, and I suspect others who share this body type have also worked hard. Would you call Queen Latifah or Oprah lazy? These extraordinary women are successful due to their work ethic, not despite their body type. The same goes for Prince Fielder, the former Detroit Tigers first baseman, and Governor Chris Christie, who both excelled in their fields. Yet, despite their success, they still face mean-spirited comments about their weight.

I recall Barbara Walters asking Governor Christie if his weight would prevent him from running for president. He responded, *"I've been working 18-hour days for my state, and I'm not slowing down."* Walters pressed further about his weight, to which he replied,

"If I knew what to do, I would do it." His words hit home and motivated me to finish this book. Christie isn't lazy or undisciplined; like many of us, he's fighting a fitness war in unfamiliar terrain. And you can't win a war if you don't understand the battlefield or the enemy.

If you're reading this, you're likely not lazy either. You've achieved success in many areas of life, but perhaps you've struggled with this one battle. We need to recognize that we're not lazy or undisciplined; we've just been fighting the wrong war with unrealistic goals, leading to frustration. But that's about to change.

Another stereotype is that endomorphs avoid discomfort and have low pain tolerance, so they don't push themselves enough to see results. But I disagree. Many endomorphs have faced rejection and ridicule for years and have built a high tolerance for both psychological and physical pain. The real challenge isn't enduring the pain — it's the frustration of seeing progress slip away after one moment of discipline failure. We must understand that our bodies require more effort to maintain fitness, and while discomfort is inevitable, perseverance, grit, and mental toughness will help us win this battle.

Research also suggests that endomorphs are calm and experience low levels of stress. While I agree that we tend to approach issues with a level head, I don't believe we experience less stress. In fact, if we don't stress enough about our physical health, we risk becoming complacent. Motivation and commitment are the foundation of any successful fitness program. If past experiences have led you to think, *"It doesn't matter what I do, I'll never reach that goal,"* you've already admitted defeat. This program will teach you to redefine success in a way that helps you achieve tangible results.

We need to stress—just a little—about the battles ahead. This is a long war, and if we don't engage emotionally, we risk slipping into complacency. It's essential to assess your motivation and energy weekly. Remember, this is your battle. Your support system can't fight it for you. You must muster the will to engage—your success is in your hands.

There's also the stereotype that endomorphs are more emotional. While showing emotion has its positives, this tends to imply that we get easily frustrated and give up. I understand the frustration of working harder than others just to achieve the same result. But while frustration is natural, so is the joy of achievement. Focus on what you can achieve, not unrealistic perfection, and avoid slipping into defeat.

Lastly, the claim that endomorphs have lower self-esteem and confidence is rooted in a lifetime of unfulfilled goals and negative feedback. If you've been told you're lazy or undisciplined, these judgments can stick. But we can win this battle by setting realistic goals and showing that while others may be genetically gifted, they aren't inherently better. Until now, you may have been striving toward an unrealistic standard based on mesomorphic ideals. It's time to set our own standards, fight hard to achieve them, and own the results.

Instead of focusing on pounds, let's shift to action-based goals. If you can improve your performance and build upon it, success will follow, and self-esteem will rise naturally. Trust me — I've been there. Tomorrow, we'll explore the positive traits of endomorphs and how to use them to your advantage.

The Good and How to Use It in our Favor

While society often critiques our endomorph bodies, it's important to note that there are also positive perceptions. Interestingly, the same people who comment on physical appearance often describe endomorphs as warmhearted, sympathetic, good-natured, and agreeable. They may even see us as more trusting (though, admittedly, this might not always work in our favor). Beyond these societal assessments, there are psychological traits linked to endomorphs that can shape our approach to fitness and wellness. Some of these traits might present hurdles, while others can become powerful assets in our journey toward success.

First, endomorphs are often seen as humorous and great with people. If this describes you, building connections within a supportive community is a natural fit. This is central to our Endomorph @ War approach. By joining together, we'll support each other through personal battles, redefine success, and raise our performance across all areas of life. Together, we'll inspire our own communities by leading the charge.

Second, endomorphs tend to be goal-oriented, which is a fantastic trait! The issue in the past may have been setting misguided goals. Now, you'll learn to focus on what's within your control and pursue those goals with determination, as if it were your job!

Lastly, endomorphs are known for their tolerance, and this trait is critical. To succeed in this battle, tolerance is non-negotiable. You'll need to push harder than others, adapt to injuries or life changes, and most importantly, accept yourself for who you are. You're an endomorph, and that's okay. By staying committed, you'll become the best version of yourself—and we'll be with you every step of the way.

Section Two: The Mental Performance Foundation – Who you Must Become.

"What you think affects how you perform. Training your brain is as important as training your body." Gary Mack

This WAR will be won on your mind first...period! When we look at the thousands of fitness programs that have been created since the 1970s such as Jazzercise, step aerobics, box fit, TRX, and CrossFit to just name a few, their success rate is linked to one thing only: **the individual's desire and motivation to stay engaged**. The same can be said for all the nutrition and diet programs such as Weight Watchers, low-fat, no-fat, no-carbs, keto, and many others, the common denominator was that the **individual was finally ready to pay the price**. Of course, after our introduction, you now know that the price will differ for each individual and for endomorphs that price is high and constant. Sadly, most people in society do not care or will ever try to understand that difference. They will make judgements based on their lack of information or willingness to understand it. But for us in the Endomorph Army, that will not matter. We will take a different approach and the only thing that will truly matter is our performance and winning our personal daily battles. The bullies, the uninformed, and the unwilling can, as it is now politically correct to say in books, *go F*ck themselves!* This is not about them; you are not doing despite them or for them, you are engaging in this battle yourself and for yours.

What is Mental Performance?

The field of exercise and sport psychology has developed over the last century and has taken many forms and names as individuals who dedicated their lives to study performance psychology had to battle against all odds for recognition as part of the general and clinical psychological community. However, we are in a time now where most organizations choose to have mental performance consultants and these organizations, for the most part, understand that mental health and wellbeing is a continuum, and that mental performance training can impact everyone's approach to life, business, academics, sports, or fitness engagement. Therefore, the foundation of this program has its roots in your understanding the inner working of your head and heart related values and how they impact your performance decisions each day. We are not engaging in a clinical relationship but one that is more of connection and mentorship. One that will allow you the opportunity to understand yourself, your thoughts, behaviors, and actions and will give you an opportunity to create new perspectives. In my experience with athletes, professionals, soldiers, and fitness participants over the last 30 years, I have identified that staying connected with your inner workings and finding creative ways to make them come alive every day is where we begin to make a difference in our approach and then see the fruits of our labor. Be advised, that a war you are about to enter is against your genetic makeup and has no deadline, it has no end state other than becoming and maintaining the best version of yourself, it is something that needs to be sustained and the only way to do that is to learn and apply principles connected to drive, competitiveness, and adaptability. In war terms, the best we are aiming for is a cease fire. To get to where we want to go and then fight like hell to sustain it. The three key components of the mental performance approach mentioned above will be the foundational triangle that will help you achieve the level of quality life that you have been searching for but your genetic make up and the nature of our thinking process has blocked you from achieving.

What are the skills and how do they relate to being an Endomorph?

The mental skills and tools that we will be working, and you will learn through the lessons and interactions with the **Endomorph @ War ™** programs are ones that can be measured and can be trained. I will do a basic summary in this book but please understand that as you commit to entering our community and program, you will receive much more detail and information about each of these areas of mental performance. First, let us describe the five mental skills and how they can impact your ability to win your daily personal battles.

Motivation - One of the three principles described above was drive. Drive is directly connected with motivation as they are somewhat connected with how badly you want something and why. For example, if your drive is connected to the external goal of fitting into a dress for the wedding you will be attending next summer, you will be fired up and motivated. You will control your cravings and will wake up to do your exercise routine. However, what happens the day after the wedding? What needs to change for you to stay on the course? Our approach to motivation needs to be different, it needs to be intrinsic because you are likely to have many falls and drawbacks along the way. As we have learned, <u>you **WILL** have to **FIGHT** and **WORK** harder than most and because of it, you will need your motivation to be steady</u>.

Composure - Emotions are part of our journey. Sadly, our society tells us daily that we need to push them away, that we need to reject them. However, I believe that we need to learn to embrace them and recognize the multiple scenarios that lead us to certain levels of emotions. For many people, endomorphs included, high level emotions lead to overeating and some other destructive behaviors. It can lead us to make irrational decisions that may work against our goals and objectives. If we can't recognize, accept, and embrace our emotions, we can't expect to win these daily battles.

Concentration - How many times you have selected a meal just because it was routine? How many times, during the previous programs, when you went to complete your journal, you did not know why you made the decisions you made in fitness and in nutrition? This is the power of concentration. We must learn and must master the ability to be in the moment. For example, genetically gifted folks can make several mistakes on their intake because of lack of focus, they will not pay the same price you will pay for making the same mistake; therefore, we must master the ability to be in the now and to give 100% of our attention at the time we are making decisions. I guarantee you that if you think about it before you do it, you will beat the odds at least 99.7% of the time.

Confidence - This is the goal of the mental game. That you walk around like you understand who you are and what you can achieve. Confidence can be seen and can be felt. Confidence is built by laying bricks in your foundation and then winning small battles every day. <u>If you learn to measure success effectively, then confidence will be something we can improve and can sustain for a long period of time</u>. Remember, even when body composition and looks are the only permissible aspect today that people can be openly disrespected and criticized in America and maybe the World, if you know who you are, if you are winning your battles, and if you are armed with what to say and the questions that you need to ask, no one, but no one, will mess with you and your mindset.

Resilience/Adaptability - If I could sell this one, I would be a millionaire! What does it take for us to stay in the fight? Yes, we already know that motivation impacts the way we stay on the course, but resilience and adaptability is where the cookie crumbles. You may want it but if you are not capable of seeing and accepting how slow progress can be your motivational fire will begin to wind down. Resilience is the stack of logs that you need to continue to throw in the fire so you can keep it alive. If you are running out of logs, then adaptability is finding paper or something else that will keep the fire going until you can cut more wood and create another stack of logs. Without resilience you can't survive this endomorph battle and that is where many people are. Many of our brothers and sisters have thrown the towel, mostly because they ran out of wood and thought that it was worthless to go get more. They were defining and measuring success wrong and there is not enough wood in the world to keep that kind of fire alive. Let us think differently, let us find strength in our community, as your peak performance coach, I have plenty of logs that I am willing to let you borrow. We can win this war together.

The next segment of this chapter will introduce you to the E@W basic mental tools. These mental tools are the strategies that you will put into play each day to win battles and to improve your mental skills.

Endomorph @ War ™ Mental Tools

The tools you will learn to use in our program can be transferred to multiple areas of your life. Once you learn them and add them to your toolbox, you own them for life, and once you master them through your application and consistency in the different levels of our program, you will have the confidence necessary to win your battles every day. There are six key tools we will use weekly as you begin to prepare, execute, and review your daily battles: goal setting, visualization, emotional energy management, self-talk, mindfulness, and the after-action review. The tools will help you improve your skills and will help you align for your war. As you plan your approach to defeat the challenges that are part of your reality, these tools will be critical for success day by day. A basic overview of these tools can be found below:

Goal Setting - The goals we set in our program will be different than those you have done in the past. We will measure success differently and we will have a battle buddy to help you stay accountable.

Visualization - Our mind is powerful, and we can create emotions and confidence by intentionally building realistic images in our mind. We will use visualization and imagery strategies to gain confidence to win the battles that we struggle with the most.

Emotional Energy Management - Understanding and developing a different relationship with our emotions is key to success in all areas of performance. We will learn to manage the situations that lead us to lose some of our personal daily battles.

Winning the Internal Conversation - In average, we have around 60,000 thoughts a day. These are internal conversations that can impact our capacity to do the actions we need to do to accomplish our goals. We need to win these internal battles to give ourselves a chance.

Mindfulness - When we are not in the moment, we miss opportunities. We will practice our capacity to focus and maximize our potential at any given moment.

Daily and Weekly Reviews - We need to develop the habit of reviewing our actions and to make the adjustments needed to stay in the fight. We can't afford to not check our progress because, unlike the other two somatotypes, we regress quickly and that leads to a negative impact on motivation.

Believing in Mottos

I am 100% convinced that phrases, quotes, and mottos can impact our mindset and by extension our actions and behaviors. For example, when I joined the Army in the 80s as a non-English speaking private, the Army's motto of the time was *"Be All You Can Be."* I believed in that motto, made it my own, and then worked my butt off to become all I could be. I embraced that phrase and made it my way of living. I hope that the motto of our program, **_"Dominate the_**

_30"_, will inspire you in a similar way. If you make peace with the idea that, as unfair as it is, YOU must pay a higher price for your fitness level and that for some fitness is war, then you will face your daily battles with a different mindset. <u>Bottom line, when it comes to fitness, YOU ARE an UNDERDOG, you must battle like one to dominate the 30% that is under your control.</u>

    Remember, as an endomorph, your genetic makeup is different. That does not preclude you from achieving your goals, I am your witness, as I have done it multiple times and in multiple settings. However, it means that you need to recognize that it will be harder for you, that it will require more work, and that you cannot take your eye off the prize or nature will remind you who is in charge. Also remember that outside of you, me, and others like you (that you will meet in our community and on this journey), NO ONE CARES. Your battles are your battles, and you cannot feel sorry for yourself or walk around upset because you were dealt a "bad hand". You need to begin acting like an underdog…you must do and sacrifice more than most to get the same results…accept it! I will be here all the way. It is a strength of mine to make underdog individuals and teams effective and turn them into champions who lead their own way. The Endomorph @ War ™ community will be no different. Life is full of successful underdogs and what they all have in common is that they know that if they wanted to experience success, <u>their route would look different than others</u>. Underdogs must do extraordinary things to give themselves a chance and they see that reality as a blessing rather than a curse because there is no better feeling than earning and achieving something you worked for. Remember, embrace your reality, and **"Dominate the 30!"**

Next chapter, we will look at the basic principles of Sun Tzu's Art of War to find inspiration for our strategy and approach. No war can be won without a plan, at this point of this journey, you have an idea what your ammunition and weapons will be. The next step is to develop the foundation of your plan.

Section Three: Why is it a War? - Planning the War: Assessments, Goal Setting, and Commitment

"Because of your genetics, you can't leave it to chance."
Dr Morales

Now that you understand what an endomorph is, the challenges that being one brings to the fitness and wellness journey, and that you have a general concept of the mental tools we will use to win our daily battles, it is time to look at why we are calling this a war. Earlier in the book, I introduced the concept of military operations throughout history where units will gain terrain and for some reason, could be resources, motivational, terrain based, etc., would lose it back forcing them to reorganize and get additional resources to re engage in the battle. At times, the unit is so demoralized that it quits and loses the war. Any of this sounds familiar? Have you personally experienced these setbacks and losses? If you are like me, I know you have. However, units that plan well, that have all the resources they need, and keep the morale of their troops up, give themselves a better chance to win. As stated during the mental performance introduction, this war will be won in the mind first, so before we plan, we need to see where we are in our motivation and drive.

Stages of Change

The "stages of change" model has been used to help individuals assess where they are in their willingness to embrace change. The model has six stages and each of them represents an area of the cycle that we are very familiar with. I am assuming that this is not the first fitness and wellness book you have picked up and that you have tried other programs in the past; therefore, you are extremely familiar with all the areas of this cycle. Just in case, here is a quick summary of each of these specific stages:

Pre-Contemplation - During this phase, you are not even aware that there is a problem. You are happy and are not even considering a change. Again, I am going to go out on a limb here and say that if you picked up a book called "For Some, Fitness is War", you are not at this stage.

Contemplation - This stage of change is where the individual is beginning to realize that some adjustments are needed. Picking up this book and the hundred other times that you considered starting a program represents this phase. You know some things may need to change.

Preparation - In this stage, the negative effects of what you considered that needed change overwhelmingly surpass the positive benefits of not doing anything about it. During this stage, you pay for the membership, you buy the new elliptical or stationary bike. You begin to plan what your new routine will be.

Action - You are now in the groove. You are sticking to your program, and you have begun to see benefits. Your new routine has become easier, and you have created some new habits. With the right motivation, we can live here for a while.

Maintenance - After you have been in the action phase for a while, your battle now becomes to maintain it. For endomorphs, this can be a very challenging phase because if you measure success in the wrong way, you will become frustrated and will lapse or relapse. Maintenance is a mental battle, is a battle of wills between you and your inner self. You must be ready and willing to pay the price to stay on this stage.

Relapse-Lapse - A lapse is a temporary failure, setback, or negative judgment call. A relapse is when you go back to what you used to be and have given up on your battles. This completes the cycle and then you must start back at the beginning. It is my opinion that you never go back to pre-contemplation. Once you have been here, once you have done it, you can be in denial but could never think that there is nothing wrong at all. At times, we endomorphs blame relapses to the lack of good programming, to not feeling like it anymore but, based on testimonials from the individuals I have worked with, it is that feeling that does not make sense to do it, that it does not matter how hard we work we can't get to the goal we want which is flawed to begin with, that takes us to relapse. I said it once and will say it again, if you were born to be an apple, be the best apple you can be. Stop trying to transform yourself to something you are not capable of sustaining. If you continue to measure success by that type of transformation, you will live in this phase of the model, and no one will be able to pull you out.

Psychological Commitment

Without commitment, we have nothing. If we are not willing to pay a higher price and make decisions based on that approach, we cannot win. As a member of the Endomorph Army ™, you will be asked to assess your commitment every day. It is a simple scale. An arrow that represents a continuum with three basic levels of commitment. This is a personal assessment, but you need to remind yourself each day how committed you will be to winning your personal battles today and why. Here are the definitions for the three areas:

I want to Quit - This is the farthest point to the left. If you are here, you don't want to continue, and you have decided that the goals you laid down during our initial stages are no longer worth pursuing.

I am Compliant - This is the middle point of the continuum. You are saying to yourself, "I will do the basics to win some easy battles." If you checked the line, you are aware of the battles that you must engage in but may let the moment get the best of you. You give yourself a 50/50 chance of winning today.

I am Obsessed - This is the farthest point to the right of the scale. You are determined to win every single battle, every decision throughout your day. You know what to do and you are obsessed about getting the results you want to get. Today, nothing will get in the way.

This daily assessment and the actual statement of your why will "recenter" you for that day and will give you motivation for the upcoming battles.

Understanding your Battlefield (Body and Fitness Related) - Based on Sun Tzu's Art War Tenets

"The art of war teaches us to rely not on the likelihood of the enemy's not coming, but on our own readiness to receive him; not on the chance of his not attacking, but rather on the fact that we have made our position unassailable." – Sun Tzu

The Art of War is one of the most read military books in the history of the world. Developed many centuries ago, it has been at the desk of every military officer and leader I have known and is studied at the highest of military tactics and education in many countries. As a former military officer, I was exposed to the Art of War as an ROTC cadet, later as a Captain at the Naval Command and Staff College, and later a much deeper dive as a Major at the Command and General Staff College in Fort Leavenworth, Kansas. The concepts presented in this book are simple but have multiple applications to several areas of military policy, tactics, and the execution of war. Since we have agreed that *For Some, Fitness is War*, it makes sense to frame some strategies and plans based on these time-proven strategies for wagging war. In this section, I will explain the basics and where these concepts fit in the program that you will be engaging as part of the *Endomorph @ War*™ Community. There are 13 basic tenets in Sun Tzu's approach, and these are the basic concepts and how they apply to our personal daily battles:

Laying Plans/Calculations - The most notable and relevant passage from this chapter states, *"The general who wins a battle makes calculations in his temple before the battle is fought."* Guess what? You are the GENERAL. You are in charge. All this tenet is trying to tell us is that without a plan, you do not have a shot. Without preparation there will be no success. We cannot expect to just show up, do the same we have always done, and then expect a different result. <u>If you know that your enemy is being hungry in the middle of the day and you don't plan for that, you will fail that day</u>. There are many more examples that we will cover in the several components of our approach, but I believe this one hits the spot.

- **Waging War -** From this tenet, I truly enjoy and try to apply the following passage *"In war, then, let your great object be victory, not lengthy campaigns."* While our battles will be lengthy because we have different challenges that most when it comes to health and wellness, our victory is redefined by winning our daily battles, by reaching the goals we set, and then by maintaining what we say is important to us. Realistic and performance-based goals will be our victory and only we will control the outcome.

  Attack by Stratagem/The Plan of Attack - This is the essence of our program. We need a strategy, we need to know what we are facing, and we need to know what to do to stay consistent in the pursuit of our realistic performance-based goals. The most applicable passage related to this tenet states as follows *"If you know the enemy and know yourself you need not fear the result of a hundred battles. If you know yourself but not the enemy for every victory gained, you also suffer a defeat. If you know neither the enemy nor yourself, you will succumb in every battle."* <u>When you know yourself and accept who you are and your challenges, then your plan can be personalized, and you give yourself a better chance to win</u>.

Tactical Dispositions - Yes! It is all about preparation. The most relevant aspect from the Sun Tzu's teachings here is that *"The skillful fighter put himself in a position which makes defeat impossible and does not miss the moment for defeating the enemy."* Once again, you need to plan ahead of time. During the early weeks on the Endomorph @ War ™ journey you will go through a process of self-discovery. On that journey, you will be able to identify how your weekly planning can set you up for success against any enemy you may encounter each of the days that week.

Energy - Sun Tzu stated, *"In battle, there are not more than two methods of attack, the direct and indirect; yet this combination gives rise to an endless series of maneuvers."*

The quote above about can be applied to a fitness and wellness journey in several ways, illustrating the need for both straightforward and creative strategies in achieving success. We can look at training and nutrition as direct methods. These are the fundamental, straightforward actions like structured workouts, balanced nutrition, proper sleep, and consistency. In fitness, the direct approach is often the disciplined execution of exercises, meal planning, and adhering to a routine. These methods are clear and necessary for progress.

Mental & lifestyle adjustments can be considered indirect actions. The indirect approach could represent the mental, emotional, and lifestyle factors that support the fitness journey. Things like mindset shifts, stress management, habit formation, and community support are less obvious but equally essential. For example, finding ways to stay motivated or adjust your environment to promote healthier choices can be indirect methods of achieving fitness goals.

Adapting & Progressing are your endless maneuvers. Just like in battle, where the combination of direct and indirect methods leads to countless maneuvers, in fitness, blending both approaches creates adaptability. You may need to change tactics — adjusting workout styles, addressing mental barriers, or finding new motivations. Combining both direct actions and creative problem-solving allows you to overcome plateaus and stay engaged.

Weak Points and Strong/Illusion and Reality: I believe that during the introduction, we addressed many of the challenges and perceived weak points in the hand that we have been dealt with. This quote from the Art of War served as an inspiration for the development of this program. The passage with the most impact here is *"Water shapes its course according to the nature of the ground over which it flows; the soldier works out his victory in relation to the foe whom he is facing."* If one of the most necessary elements chooses its movement based on and around the natural landscape that exists, why can't we do the same. We must work around what we have been given. We need to find a way to succeed.

Maneuvering: Ponder and deliberate before you make a move. As endomorphs, we are challenged throughout our day and are constantly putting out fires and engaging in personal decisions. Plan your day, your routes, and your activities to work around the things that will challenge you the most. Have a plan for the times you will face adversity and maneuver around.

Variation in Tactics: "*There are roads that must not be followed.*" As you embark on your self-discovery journey, you will learn that there are things you do not enjoy and you must learn to design a program that will fit your personality and, at times, it is wise to have multiple options for each area of development. This will keep you from boredom and will help you stay in the fight.

The Army on the March/Moving the Force: "*After crossing the river, you should get far away from it.*" This program is designed to help you identify the things that get in the way and replace them with more realistic possibilities. If something starts working for us, we do not deliberately drop it because we now feel good, we make it part of our approach. We will keep moving forward, first leading yourself and then taking your fight to the world.

Terrain/Situational Positioning: *"Looks at the three general areas of resistance (distance, dangers, and barriers) and the six types of ground positions that arise from them. Each of these six field positions offer certain advantages and disadvantages."* We have already studied some of the obstacles that are common to all of us, but we will learn to identify our personal obstacles as well. Each of us has a different environment, we must know the terrain we are working on and have a plan for it.

The Nine Situations/Nine Terrains: *"When a chieftain is fighting in his own territory, it is dispersive ground."* Military leaders understand how multiple variable and different situations can affect the outcome of their battle. They study meticulously where they can be trapped and where they are vulnerable. We will identify areas of our life in which modification must be made for us to have a better chance at reaching our goals.

The Attack by Fire: *"Explains the general use of weapons and the specific use of the environment as a weapon."* We are definitively going on the attack. This program is called Endomorph at War for a reason, we are going change our mindsets towards fitness and wellness, we are going to use performance as our target, and we are going to use our new confidence to change our environments.

The Use of Spies/Use of Intelligence: *"Focuses on the importance of developing good information sources and specifies the five types of intelligence sources and how to best manage each of them."* Every week of the program you will receive the best information available through the lenses of an endomorph. I will be your spy, your intelligence (information) source. Over the last decade, I have read every book about obesity, nutrition, and how the body react differently based on nutrient content and your body chemistry. You will be armed and ready.

Section Four: Fitness Foundations through the Endomorph's Eyes - Endomorph Soldier's Rules of Engagement

So, you have some physical and genetics-based challenges...now what? We must now prepare a personalized program that has a foundation based on exercise principles and that will help you better define what this battle will be for you. To this, you must start with a basic understanding of why we must look at the fitness information available from the lenses of an endomorph.

As part of this community, we will do this via video lessons and weekly live seminars where you will have an opportunity to challenge the status quo with your own experiences. My approach is to teach you what the exercise science concepts are, analyze where we need to challenge and emphasize based on our needs, and finally create a program that you can take ownership of. No more mandated this or that, no more canned programs, you will have the choice. You will assess yourself, identify your strengths and areas for improvement, and you will create something that works for you and circumstances. After that, you will take that plan to the world. Below are some of the key elements you will be exposed during the first 12 weeks on the E@W community's educational and performance journey:

- *Components of Fitness and how to assess yourself.*
- *Principles of Exercise and how to use them to ensure program success.*
- *Endomorphs and Physical Activity: The key to turn your metabolism around.*
- *How to create an unbreakable contract with yourself.*
- *Connecting your Motivation to Exercise to a Bigger Picture.*
- *Elements of Personalized Goal Setting: The Endomorph's Best Friend*
- *Individualized personal assessment based on family and reality...not media, friends, etc.*
- *Strategies to Implement Physical Activity into a Busy Schedule*

Section Five: Endomorphs and Nutrition

Here is where many of our frustrations live. As endomorphs, we see everyone else around us enjoying the same foods we enjoy and paying no price for indiscretions. This is where we get angry and begin to search for a quick solution and where the diet and exercise business world has made the most of its earnings. Hundreds of programs have been created, marketed, and sold with the promise that there will be change, that this time will be different. As previously stated, I have spent the last 15 years reading and researching all these programs, books, and many "get there quick" type schemes. The conclusion is clear, and widely reported: diets do not work! The industry has no common standard on how they report their results. They can pick and choose how they write their findings and most of the time they do it in a confusing manner that will market to a small group of the population but will make great claims. Here is one of the latest examples. Recently, the diet industry began reporting the effectiveness of apple cider vinegar as a great weight loss product. In their advertisement they would say, *"people lost weight after taking this supplement early in the morning."* This statement is correct but at the same time, while it makes business sense to say this, the reality is that based on research, the only people who lost weight using this supplement were the ones who got nauseous and felt sick after taking it in the morning and therefore did not eat well during the rest of the day. Some may say, *"well, if feeling a bit sick and losing your appetite is the price that I must pay for losing a couple of pounds, then so be it."* However, this is not the way it has to be. Science shows the power of genetics and how your body will react to food, and in our community, you will learn to see food differently, understand how to make better selections, and most importantly how to define success the right way in this area of your personal battle.

The last three books I have read about dealing with obesity, eating, the realities of diets, and the inner workings of the diet and fitness "industry" all had these three things in common. First, they shared the studies conducted on identical twins separated at birth who were exposed to two different environments growing and how much alike their body composition still was as adults regardless of how fit and active their adoptive parents were. Second, these books all spoke about the combination of diet and exercise as the key to accomplishing goals in this area. Lastly, diets do not have a long shelf life. They alter who we are and what we like to do. We can do them for a short period of time, to reach an important temporary goal but they are not sustainable. The solution is not to throw your hands in the air and quit, as many do because of the frustration. The solution is to engage in this daily battle and win every engagement. We have already established that you will be hungry, you cannot change that. However, you can win on timing and decisions. You can win by being aware of your selections and by preparing ahead of time. You can also win by accepting that you must be **"Willing to Pay a Higher Price"** for your health and wellness and that you must **"Dominate the 30."** Not for your appearance, not for show, but for performance.

Here are some of the key topics you will be exposed during your educational journey as part of the E@W Community and all through the lenses of an endomorph:

- *Why diets do not work.*

- *Macronutrients and how they help or hinder the endomorphs' metabolism.*
- *Micronutrients and how they help or hinder the endomorphs' metabolism.*
- *Hydration and Electrolytes Balance*
- *Making your meal plans.*
- *Strategies for winning your daily battles in fueling and nutrition.*

Section Six: Dominate the 30 - Endomorph @ War Rules of Engagement for Fitness and Nutrition

What does Dominate the 30 Mean?

About 70% of our body is influenced by genetics while 30% is under our control and this relates to the interaction between genetics (heredity) and environmental factors (lifestyle). This concept is commonly referenced in discussions about epigenetics and nature vs. nurture debates.

Genetics play a significant role in determining aspects of our physical structure and metabolic processes, accounting for around 70% of traits like body type, muscle fiber composition, metabolism, and even susceptibility to diseases. For example, as previously discussed, people are born with a general body type—endomorph, mesomorph, or ectomorph—which dictates tendencies toward storing fat, muscle development, or being lean. In addition, an individual's basal metabolic rate (BMR), which affects how quickly you burn calories at rest, is largely genetic. Some people are predisposed to faster or slower metabolism. Lastly, conditions like obesity, diabetes, and cardiovascular diseases have strong genetic links, making some people more prone to these conditions regardless of lifestyle choices.

The remaining 30% is influenced by choices we make, such as:

- Diet and Nutrition: What we eat directly impacts weight, muscle gain, and overall health. Nutritional choices can optimize or hinder our genetic potential.
- Physical Activity: Exercise can help manage weight, improve cardiovascular health, and enhance muscle growth, regardless of one's genetic predisposition.
- Stress and Sleep: How well you manage stress and how much sleep you get can affect your body's response to training and overall health.

These facts can be found in literature and empirical studies in the field of epigenetics which is the study of how gene expression is influenced by environmental factors. While the DNA sequence remains unchanged, lifestyle factors can switch genes on or off, influencing things like fat storage, metabolism, and cellular repair.

While genetics set a framework for our body composition and health, lifestyle choices have the power to modify the expression of these genes. A proper diet, exercise, and other healthy habits can optimize the 30% of variables we control, potentially reducing the impact of unfavorable genetic predispositions.

Because of these factors, we must engage in a series of personal battles that can help us maximize the things that we can control. These rules are described below for your review and implementation.

The E@W Rules

As part of your journey, we will discuss basic strategies to help you win every day. Consistency of effort helps define the level of success you will have in the long run in your personal war against your genetics. During week one of your level one program, you will be provided more details behind the why for these 10 E@W Rules, but in general they are designed to give you a compass for your daily interactions and personal assessments. These are strategies I have used effectively in my life but when I took my eyes from them or chose to ignore them, it all went back to normal, to the status quo dictated by my genetic composition. Again, as you move from level one to level two, you will begin to have flexibility in personalizing and adjusting these based on your personal challenges. Our foundational approach includes the following daily strategies:

1. Eat for Fuel not for joy for the majority of your meals (change your relationship with food).

2. Stay on Calorie Limit (ex. 2,500 on Workout Days and 2,000 on non-Workout Days depending on your personal needs.)

3. Lightest Meal before 2 hours before bedtime (u500)

4. Drink Water when Extremely Hungry.

5. No drinking your calories unless is a protein shake acting as a meal.

6. Follow YOUR physical activity schedule. Do at least 30 minutes of physical activity daily.

7. Weigh in only on Tuesday and Friday mornings; however, place more value on performance than the scale.

8. If diabetes is in your genetic line, check for blood glucose and insulin control; limit your carb intake. Aim to eat less than 150g from Monday to Saturday during Level 1 Training.

9. ADD YOUR personal challenge # 1 here _____.

10. ADD YOUR personal challenge # 2 here _____.

You will understand the why for all of these and have the opportunity after several weeks of personal assessments to personalize your own two rules.

Section Seven: Joining the E@W Army Community

Intrigued yet? Are some of these things starting to make sense to you based on your personal experiences? If so, I think you are ready to join us on this journey. Our community has been designed to become a worldwide movement that will help us understand that there are many more out there who face the same challenges. Through this community, we want to show that there is strength in numbers that if we support each other, we can win these battles and we can even influence others to begin to win theirs. Our community lives online, but we will be family. We will be a team that is spread out throughout the world, and we will know when we cross paths with each other because we will handle ourselves with confidence. People will be able to tell that you measure up too much more than what the eye can see. If you are ready, visit our website now at www.peakmentalgame.com/communities and enroll in the next course. We start a new cohort each Monday and look forward to seeing you there. Let us win this war together.

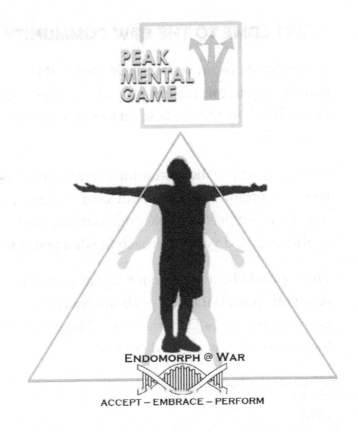

E@W LEVEL ONE JOURNAL

KNOW YOURSELF, LOVE YOURSELF, LEAD YOURSELF

"Willing to PAY a Higher Price"

NAME: _____

LEVEL ONE COHORT: _____

WELCOME TO THE E@W COMMUNITY

Congratulations on your decision to get this journal, to join this community, and to challenge yourself to become the best version of you that you can be.

I look forward to the community interactions but most importantly to hear about your success and how your mindset is impacting your life, your confidence, and your approach to what you do.

There should be no reason for any of us not to reach our potential if our goals are based on performance. Let's Dominate the 30 together over the next twelve weeks and beyond.

Yours in the battle,

DrM

The Mental Skills Coach in your Back Pocket!

SUCCESS MAP EXAMPLE

Hector R. Morales-Negron, PhD, CMPC, ACSM-PT
Lieutenant Colonel, USA (R)
2021 Fitness Blueprint
Army Master Fitness Trainer, Army Master Combatives Instructor
Founder of MORALES Dojo – ENDOMORPH AT WAR (E@W)

DrM's WHY
To BE: A Warrior Mindset Builder, A Developer of the Competitive Edge, Lens Changer and Fitness Perspective Creation Magician. Through my example, change the definition of success to one that is performance.

SIGNATURE STRENGHTS
- Passion – Reflected in all I do and in all my interactions.
- Loyalty – To my team, my family, and my passions.
- EQ – To modify my approach to leadership and to meet everyone at their starting point without judgment.
- Creativity in Communications – Always finding a way to get the message across.

FITNESS Core Convictions
- Fitness is More Difficult for Some – Genetics is powerful. Some must sacrifice more for the same result.
- Looks CAN'T Outweigh Performance – Stop being satisfied with JUST creating goals based on looks. Think performance, value achievement above the superficial.
- Fitness Can't Be Achieved On Your Own – We are our best when we are accountable to others.
- Fitness is a Head and Heart Matter – Exercise Psychology Fundamentals are Critical.

FITNESS VISION for 2021

AS Program Developer
Create a program that is inclusive, and everyone can achieve performance in their own journey. Provide opportunities for people to succeed.

As a Man
<u>Be prepared for the unexpected</u>. Return to your physical performance roots. People are using things you created, you have more experience and passion that most. Return to retirement physical condition by year end and to Pre-Korea status by Jun 2020.

Obstacles and Plans to Defeat Them
Genetics (Don't take days off)
Constant Hunger (plan for it)
Work Requirements (Find the Way)
Retirement Mentality (Screw Retirement – Live)

MY WORD FOR 2021
OBSESSED

YOUR LEVEL 1 SUCCESS MAP

What is your why?

Name your Top Three Signature Strengths

1.

2.

3.

Based on your Level One experience, what are your Top Three Fitness Convictions?

1.

2.

3.

What is your vision for this program?

Top Three Obstacles (Work Around)

1.

2.

3.

WORD FOR THIS 20 Weeks:

GOALS FOR THIS PROGRAM

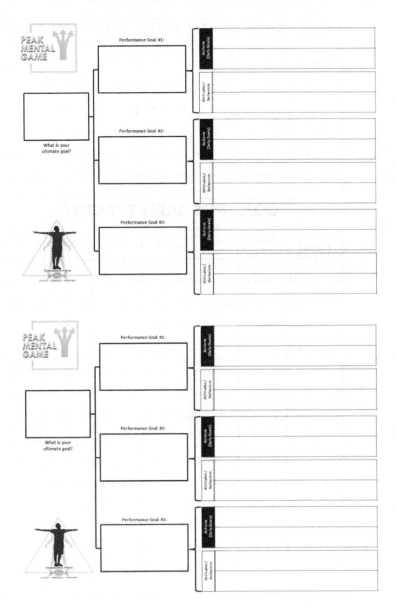

Week One Matrix

SUN	MON	TUE	WED	THU	FRI	SAT

GOAL PROGRESS TRACKER

Goal	Date	Date	Date	Date	Date	Date

DAILY FITNESS TRACKER

Week One – Day 1 – DATE: _____

Today's MSE GOAL – Upper – Lower – Core – HITT

Cardio

Activity	Minutes	Level/Speed Intensity	Heart Rate	Calories Burned	Notes

Strength

Exercise	SET 1 WT/REP	SET 2 WT/REP	SET 3 WT/REP	SET 4 WT/REP	Remarks

Stretching/Mobility

Activity/Move	REPS/TIME	Notes

| ENDOMORPH @ WAR |
| LEVEL 1 – DAILY COMMITMENT |

| QUIT WHY? | COMPLIANT | OBSSESSED |

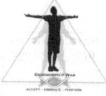

ENDOMORPH @ WAR
LEVEL ONE - DAILY REVIEW
DAILY RULES OF ENGAGEMENT

DATE_____

Today's Weight _____ BG (Tue/Fri) _____ BP _____

- ☐ Do something physical today 30+ minutes.
- ☐ Limit Carbs to less than 175 a day
- ☐ Don't drink your calories.
- ☐ Eat for Fuel, not for joy (change your relationship with food)
- ☐ Stay under 2,500 on workout days and U2K on non-workout days
- ☐ Kept the Fitness Schedule

Notes on Daily Battle:
_____
_____

FOOD INTAKE
Total Calories _____ Carbs % ____ Protein % ____ Fat % ____

NOTES ON TODAY'S NUTRITION
_____
_____

How do you qualify your day? W ____ L ____

What went well? UPS

What did not go well? What is the plan to improve it tomorrow?

What did you learn about yourself today?

DAILY FITNESS TRACKER

Week One – Day 2 – DATE: _____

Today's MSE GOAL – Upper – Lower – Core – HITT

Cardio

Activity	Minutes	Level/Speed Intensity	Heart Rate	Calories Burned	Notes

Strength

Exercise	SET 1 WT/REP	SET 2 WT/REP	SET 3 WT/REP	SET 4 WT/REP	Remarks

Stretching/Mobility

Activity/Move	REPS/TIME	Notes

ENDOMORPH @ WAR		
LEVEL 1 – DAILY COMMITMENT		
QUIT	COMPLIANT	OBSSESSED
WHY?		

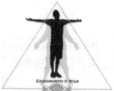

ENDOMORPH @ WAR
LEVEL ONE - DAILY REVIEW
DAILY RULES OF ENGAGEMENT

DATE_____

Today's Weight _____ BG (Tue/Fri) _____ BP _____

- ☐ Do something physical today 30+ minutes.
- ☐ Limit Carbs to less than 175 a day
- ☐ Don't drink your calories.
- ☐ Eat for Fuel, not for joy (change your relationship with food)
- ☐ Stay under 2,500 on workout days and U2K on non-workout days
- ☐ Kept the Fitness Schedule

Notes on Daily Battle:
_____
_____

FOOD INTAKE
Total Calories _____ Carbs % ____ Protein % ____ Fat % ____

NOTES ON TODAY'S NUTRITION
_____
_____
_____

How do you qualify your day? W ____ L ____

What went well? UPS

What did not go well? What is the plan to improve it tomorrow?

What did you learn about yourself today?

DAILY FITNESS TRACKER

Week One – Day 3 – DATE: _____

Today's MSE GOAL – Upper – Lower – Core – HITT

Cardio

Activity	Minutes	Level/Speed Intensity	Heart Rate	Calories Burned	Notes

Strength

Exercise	SET 1 WT/REP	SET 2 WT/REP	SET 3 WT/REP	SET 4 WT/REP	Remarks

Stretching/Mobility

Activity/Move	REPS/TIME	Notes

ENDOMORPH @ WAR
LEVEL 1 — DAILY COMMITMENT

QUIT — WHY?   COMPLIANT   OBSSESSED

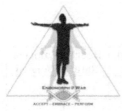

ENDOMORPH @ WAR
LEVEL ONE - DAILY REVIEW
DAILY RULES OF ENGAGEMENT

DATE_____

Today's Weight _____ BG (Tue/Fri)_____ BP _____

- ☐ Do something physical today 30+ minutes.
- ☐ Limit Carbs to less than 175 a day
- ☐ Don't drink your calories.
- ☐ Eat for Fuel, not for joy (change your relationship with food)
- ☐ Stay under 2,500 on workout days and U2K on non-workout days
- ☐ Kept the Fitness Schedule

Notes on Daily Battle;
_____
_____

FOOD INTAKE
Total Calories _____ Carbs % ____ Protein % ____ Fat % ____

NOTES ON TODAY'S NUTRITION
_____
_____
_____

How do you qualify your day? W ____ L ____

What went well? UPS

What did not go well? What is the plan to improve it tomorrow?

What did you learn about yourself today?

DAILY FITNESS TRACKER

Week One – Day 4 – DATE: _____

Today's MSE GOAL – Upper – Lower – Core – HITT

Cardio

Activity	Minutes	Level/Speed Intensity	Heart Rate	Calories Burned	Notes

Strength

Exercise	SET 1 WT/REP	SET 2 WT/REP	SET 3 WT/REP	SET 4 WT/REP	Remarks

Stretching/Mobility

Activity/Move	REPS/TIME	Notes

ENDOMORPH @ WAR
LEVEL 1 — DAILY COMMITMENT

QUIT   COMPLIANT   OBSSESSED
WHY?

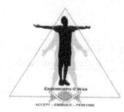

ENDOMORPH @ WAR
LEVEL ONE - DAILY REVIEW
DAILY RULES OF ENGAGEMENT

DATE_____

Today's Weight _____ BG (Tue/Fri) _____ BP _____

- ☐ Do something physical today 30+ minutes.
- ☐ Limit Carbs to less than 175 a day
- ☐ Don't drink your calories.
- ☐ Eat for Fuel, not for joy (change your relationship with food)
- ☐ Stay under 2,500 on workout days and U2K on non-workout days
- ☐ Kept the Fitness Schedule

Notes on Daily Battle:
_____
_____

FOOD INTAKE
Total Calories _____ Carbs % ____ Protein % ____ Fat % ____

NOTES ON TODAY'S NUTRITION
_____
_____
_____

How do you qualify your day? W ____ L ____

What went well? UPS

What did not go well? What is the plan to improve it tomorrow?

What did you learn about yourself today?

DAILY FITNESS TRACKER

Week One – Day 5 – DATE: _____

Today's MSE GOAL – Upper – Lower – Core – HITT

Cardio

Activity	Minutes	Level/Speed Intensity	Heart Rate	Calories Burned	Notes

Strength

Exercise	SET 1 WT/REP	SET 2 WT/REP	SET 3 WT/REP	SET 4 WT/REP	Remarks

Stretching/Mobility

Activity/Move	REPS/TIME	Notes

ENDOMORPH @ WAR
LEVEL 1 — DAILY COMMITMENT

QUIT — COMPLIANT — OBSSESSED

WHY?

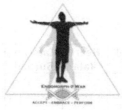

ENDOMORPH @ WAR
LEVEL ONE - DAILY REVIEW
DAILY RULES OF ENGAGEMENT

DATE_____

Today's Weight _____ BG (Tue/Fri) _____ BP _____

- ☐ Do something physical today 30+ minutes.
- ☐ Limit Carbs to less than 175 a day
- ☐ Don't drink your calories.
- ☐ Eat for Fuel, not for joy (change your relationship with food)
- ☐ Stay under 2,500 on workout days and U2K on non-workout days
- ☐ Kept the Fitness Schedule

Notes on Daily Battle:
_____
_____

FOOD INTAKE
Total Calories _____ Carbs % ____ Protein % ____ Fat % ____

NOTES ON TODAY'S NUTRITION
_____
_____
_____

How do you qualify your day? W ____ L ____

What went well? UPS

What did not go well? What is the plan to improve it tomorrow?

What did you learn about yourself today?

DAILY FITNESS TRACKER

Week One – Day 6 – DATE: _____

Today's MSE GOAL – Upper – Lower – Core – HITT

Cardio

Activity	Minutes	Level/Speed Intensity	Heart Rate	Calories Burned	Notes

Strength

Exercise	SET 1 WT/REP	SET 2 WT/REP	SET 3 WT/REP	SET 4 WT/REP	Remarks

Stretching/Mobility

Activity/Move	REPS/TIME	Notes

ENDOMORPH @ WAR
LEVEL 1 – DAILY COMMITMENT

QUIT — COMPLIANT — OBSSESSED
WHY?

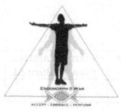

ENDOMORPH @ WAR
LEVEL ONE - DAILY REVIEW

DAILY RULES OF ENGAGEMENT

DATE_____

Today's Weight _____ BG (Tue/Fri) _____ BP _____

- ☐ Do something physical today 30+ minutes.
- ☐ Limit Carbs to less than 175 a day
- ☐ Don't drink your calories.
- ☐ Eat for Fuel, not for joy (change your relationship with food)
- ☐ Stay under 2,500 on workout days and U2K on non-workout days
- ☐ Kept the Fitness Schedule

Notes on Daily Battle;
_____
_____

FOOD INTAKE
Total Calories _____ Carbs % ____ Protein % ____ Fat % ____

NOTES ON TODAY'S NUTRITION
_____
_____
_____

How do you qualify your day? W ____ L ____

What went well? UPS

What did not go well? What is the plan to improve it tomorrow?

What did you learn about yourself today?

Week One Notes

Week Two Matrix

SUN	MON	TUE	WED	THU	FRI	SAT

GOAL PROGRESS TRACKER

Goal	Date	Date	Date	Date	Date	Date

DAILY FITNESS TRACKER

Week Two – Day 1 – DATE: _____

Today's MSE GOAL – Upper – Lower – Core – HITT

Cardio

Activity	Minutes	Level/Speed Intensity	Heart Rate	Calories Burned	Notes

Strength

Exercise	SET 1 WT/REP	SET 2 WT/REP	SET 3 WT/REP	SET 4 WT/REP	Remarks

Stretching/Mobility

Activity/Move	REPS/TIME	Notes

| ENDOMORPH @ WAR |
| LEVEL 1 – DAILY COMMITMENT |

QUIT WHY? — COMPLIANT — OBSSESSED

ENDOMORPH @ WAR
LEVEL ONE - DAILY REVIEW
DAILY RULES OF ENGAGEMENT

DATE _____

Today's Weight _____ BG (Tue/Fri) _____ BP _____

- ☐ Do something physical today 30+ minutes.
- ☐ Limit Carbs to less than 175 a day
- ☐ Don't drink your calories.
- ☐ Eat for Fuel, not for joy (change your relationship with food)
- ☐ Stay under 2,500 on workout days and U2K on non-workout days
- ☐ Kept the Fitness Schedule

Notes on Daily Battle:
_____
_____

FOOD INTAKE
Total Calories _____ Carbs % ____ Protein % ____ Fat % ____

NOTES ON TODAY'S NUTRITION
_____
_____
_____

How do you qualify your day? W ____ L ____

What went well? UPS

What did not go well? What is the plan to improve it tomorrow?

What did you learn about yourself today?

DAILY FITNESS TRACKER

Week Two – Day 2 – DATE: _____

Today's MSE GOAL – Upper – Lower – Core – HITT

Cardio

Activity	Minutes	Level/Speed Intensity	Heart Rate	Calories Burned	Notes

Strength

Exercise	SET 1 WT/REP	SET 2 WT/REP	SET 3 WT/REP	SET 4 WT/REP	Remarks

Stretching/Mobility

Activity/Move	REPS/TIME	Notes

ENDOMORPH @ WAR
LEVEL 1 – DAILY COMMITMENT

QUIT	COMPLIANT	OBSSESSED
WHY?		

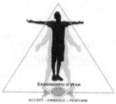

ENDOMORPH @ WAR
LEVEL ONE - DAILY REVIEW
DAILY RULES OF ENGAGEMENT

DATE_____

Today's Weight _____ BG (Tue/Fri) _____ BP _____

- ☐ Do something physical today 30+ minutes.
- ☐ Limit Carbs to less than 175 a day
- ☐ Don't drink your calories.
- ☐ Eat for Fuel, not for joy (change your relationship with food)
- ☐ Stay under 2,500 on workout days and U2K on non-workout days
- ☐ Kept the Fitness Schedule

Notes on Daily Battle:
_____
_____

FOOD INTAKE
Total Calories _____ Carbs % ____ Protein % ____ Fat % ____

NOTES ON TODAY'S NUTRITION
_____
_____
_____

How do you qualify your day? W ____ L ____

What went well? UPS

What did not go well? What is the plan to improve it tomorrow?

What did you learn about yourself today?

DAILY FITNESS TRACKER

Week Two – Day 3 – DATE: _____

Today's MSE GOAL – Upper – Lower – Core – HITT

Cardio

Activity	Minutes	Level/Speed Intensity	Heart Rate	Calories Burned	Notes

Strength

Exercise	SET 1 WT/REP	SET 2 WT/REP	SET 3 WT/REP	SET 4 WT/REP	Remarks

Stretching/Mobility

Activity/Move	REPS/TIME	Notes

ENDOMORPH @ WAR
LEVEL 1 — DAILY COMMITMENT

QUIT　　　　　　　　　COMPLIANT　　　　　　　　　OBSSESSED
WHY?

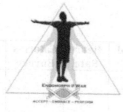

ENDOMORPH @ WAR
LEVEL ONE - DAILY REVIEW

DAILY RULES OF ENGAGEMENT

DATE_____

Today's Weight _____ BG (Tue/Fri) _____ BP _____

- ☐ Do something physical today 30+ minutes.
- ☐ Limit Carbs to less than 175 a day
- ☐ Don't drink your calories.
- ☐ Eat for Fuel, not for joy (change your relationship with food)
- ☐ Stay under 2,500 on workout days and U2K on non-workout days
- ☐ Kept the Fitness Schedule

Notes on Daily Battle:
_____
_____

FOOD INTAKE
Total Calories _____ Carbs % ____ Protein % ____ Fat % ____

NOTES ON TODAY'S NUTRITION
_____
_____
_____

How do you qualify your day? W ____ L ____

What went well? UPS

What did not go well? What is the plan to improve it tomorrow?

What did you learn about yourself today?

DAILY FITNESS TRACKER

Week Two – Day 4 – DATE: _____

Today's MSE GOAL – Upper – Lower – Core – HITT

Cardio

Activity	Minutes	Level/Speed Intensity	Heart Rate	Calories Burned	Notes

Strength

Exercise	SET 1 WT/REP	SET 2 WT/REP	SET 3 WT/REP	SET 4 WT/REP	Remarks

Stretching/Mobility

Activity/Move	REPS/TIME	Notes

ENDOMORPH @ WAR
LEVEL 1 – DAILY COMMITMENT

QUIT	COMPLIANT	OBSSESSED
WHY?		

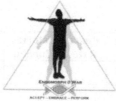

ENDOMORPH @ WAR
LEVEL ONE - DAILY REVIEW
DAILY RULES OF ENGAGEMENT

DATE_____

Today's Weight _____ BG (Tue/Fri) _____ BP _____

- ☐ Do something physical today 30+ minutes.
- ☐ Limit Carbs to less than 175 a day
- ☐ Don't drink your calories.
- ☐ Eat for Fuel, not for joy (change your relationship with food)
- ☐ Stay under 2,500 on workout days and U2K on non-workout days
- ☐ Kept the Fitness Schedule

Notes on Daily Battle:
_____
_____

FOOD INTAKE
Total Calories _____ Carbs % ____ Protein % ____ Fat % ____

NOTES ON TODAY'S NUTRITION
_____
_____
_____

How do you qualify your day? W ____ L ____

What went well? UPS

What did not go well? What is the plan to improve it tomorrow?

What did you learn about yourself today?

DAILY FITNESS TRACKER

Week Two – Day 5 – DATE: _____

Today's MSE GOAL – Upper – Lower – Core – HITT

Cardio

Activity	Minutes	Level/Speed Intensity	Heart Rate	Calories Burned	Notes

Strength

Exercise	SET 1 WT/REP	SET 2 WT/REP	SET 3 WT/REP	SET 4 WT/REP	Remarks

Stretching/Mobility

Activity/Move	REPS/TIME	Notes

ENDOMORPH @ WAR
LEVEL 1 – DAILY COMMITMENT

QUIT   COMPLIANT   OBSSESSED

WHY?

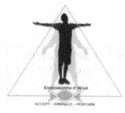

ENDOMORPH @ WAR
LEVEL ONE - DAILY REVIEW
DAILY RULES OF ENGAGEMENT

DATE_____

Today's Weight _____ BG (Tue/Fri)_____ BP _____

- ☐ Do something physical today 30+ minutes.
- ☐ Limit Carbs to less than 175 a day
- ☐ Don't drink your calories.
- ☐ Eat for Fuel, not for joy (change your relationship with food)
- ☐ Stay under 2,500 on workout days and U2K on non-workout days
- ☐ Kept the Fitness Schedule

Notes on Daily Battle:
_____
_____

FOOD INTAKE
Total Calories _____ Carbs % ___ Protein % ___ Fat % ___

NOTES ON TODAY'S NUTRITION
_____
_____
_____

How do you qualify your day? W ___ L ___

What went well? UPS

What did not go well? What is the plan to improve it tomorrow?

What did you learn about yourself today?

DAILY FITNESS TRACKER

Week Two – Day 6 – DATE: _____

Today's MSE GOAL – Upper – Lower – Core – HITT

Cardio

Activity	Minutes	Level/Speed Intensity	Heart Rate	Calories Burned	Notes

Strength

Exercise	SET 1 WT/REP	SET 2 WT/REP	SET 3 WT/REP	SET 4 WT/REP	Remarks

Stretching/Mobility

Activity/Move	REPS/TIME	Notes

ENDOMORPH @ WAR
LEVEL 1 – DAILY COMMITMENT

QUIT   COMPLIANT   OBSSESSED
WHY?

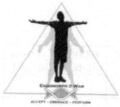

ENDOMORPH @ WAR
LEVEL ONE - DAILY REVIEW
DAILY RULES OF ENGAGEMENT
DATE_____

Today's Weight _____ BG (Tue/Fri) _____ BP _____

- ☐ Do something physical today 30+ minutes.
- ☐ Limit Carbs to less than 175 a day
- ☐ Don't drink your calories.
- ☐ Eat for Fuel, not for joy (change your relationship with food)
- ☐ Stay under 2,500 on workout days and U2K on non-workout days
- ☐ Kept the Fitness Schedule

Notes on Daily Battle:
_____
_____

FOOD INTAKE
Total Calories _____ Carbs % ____ Protein % ____ Fat % ____

NOTES ON TODAY'S NUTRITION
_____
_____
_____

How do you qualify your day? W ____ L ____

What went well? UPS

What did not go well? What is the plan to improve it tomorrow?

What did you learn about yourself today?

Week Two Notes

Week Three Matrix

SUN	MON	TUE	WED	THU	FRI	SAT

GOAL PROGRESS TRACKER

Goal	Date	Date	Date	Date	Date	Date

DAILY FITNESS TRACKER

Week Three – Day 1 – DATE: _____

Today's MSE GOAL – Upper – Lower – Core – HITT

Cardio

Activity	Minutes	Level/Speed Intensity	Heart Rate	Calories Burned	Notes

Strength

Exercise	SET 1 WT/REP	SET 2 WT/REP	SET 3 WT/REP	SET 4 WT/REP	Remarks

Stretching/Mobility

Activity/Move	REPS/TIME	Notes

ENDOMORPH @ WAR
LEVEL 1 – DAILY COMMITMENT

QUIT WHY? — COMPLIANT — OBSSESSED

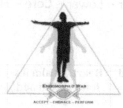

ENDOMORPH @ WAR
LEVEL ONE - DAILY REVIEW

DAILY RULES OF ENGAGEMENT

DATE _____

Today's Weight _____ BG (Tue/Fri) _____ BP _____

- ☐ Do something physical today 30+ minutes.
- ☐ Limit Carbs to less than 175 a day
- ☐ Don't drink your calories.
- ☐ Eat for Fuel, not for joy (change your relationship with food)
- ☐ Stay under 2,500 on workout days and U2K on non-workout days
- ☐ Kept the Fitness Schedule

Notes on Daily Battle:
_____
_____

FOOD INTAKE
Total Calories _____ Carbs % _____ Protein % _____ Fat % _____

NOTES ON TODAY'S NUTRITION
_____
_____
_____

How do you qualify your day? W _____ L _____

What went well? UPS

What did not go well? What is the plan to improve it tomorrow?

What did you learn about yourself today?

DAILY FITNESS TRACKER

Week Three – Day 2 – DATE: _____

Today's MSE GOAL – Upper – Lower – Core – HITT

Cardio

Activity	Minutes	Level/Speed Intensity	Heart Rate	Calories Burned	Notes

Strength

Exercise	SET 1 WT/REP	SET 2 WT/REP	SET 3 WT/REP	SET 4 WT/REP	Remarks

Stretching/Mobility

Activity/Move	REPS/TIME	Notes

ENDOMORPH @ WAR
LEVEL 1 – DAILY COMMITMENT

QUIT   COMPLIANT   OBSSESSED
WHY?

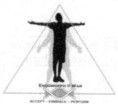

ENDOMORPH @ WAR
LEVEL ONE - DAILY REVIEW
DAILY RULES OF ENGAGEMENT
DATE_____

Today's Weight _____ BG (Tue/Fri) _____ BP _____

- ☐ Do something physical today 30+ minutes.
- ☐ Limit Carbs to less than 175 a day
- ☐ Don't drink your calories.
- ☐ Eat for Fuel, not for joy (change your relationship with food)
- ☐ Stay under 2,500 on workout days and U2K on non-workout days
- ☐ Kept the Fitness Schedule

Notes on Daily Battle:
_____
_____

FOOD INTAKE
Total Calories _____ Carbs % ____ Protein % ____ Fat % ____

NOTES ON TODAY'S NUTRITION
_____
_____
_____

How do you qualify your day? W ____ L ____

What went well? UPS

What did not go well? What is the plan to improve it tomorrow?

What did you learn about yourself today?

DAILY FITNESS TRACKER

Week Three – Day 3 – DATE: _____

Today's MSE GOAL – Upper – Lower – Core – HITT

Cardio

Activity	Minutes	Level/Speed Intensity	Heart Rate	Calories Burned	Notes

Strength

Exercise	SET 1 WT/REP	SET 2 WT/REP	SET 3 WT/REP	SET 4 WT/REP	Remarks

Stretching/Mobility

Activity/Move	REPS/TIME	Notes

ENDOMORPH @ WAR
LEVEL 1 – DAILY COMMITMENT

QUIT   COMPLIANT   OBSSESSED

WHY?

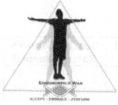

ENDOMORPH @ WAR
LEVEL ONE - DAILY REVIEW
DAILY RULES OF ENGAGEMENT

DATE_____

Today's Weight _____ BG (Tue/Fri)_____ BP _____

- ☐ Do something physical today 30+ minutes.
- ☐ Limit Carbs to less than 175 a day
- ☐ Don't drink your calories.
- ☐ Eat for Fuel, not for joy (change your relationship with food)
- ☐ Stay under 2,500 on workout days and U2K on non-workout days
- ☐ Kept the Fitness Schedule

Notes on Daily Battle:
_____
_____

FOOD INTAKE
Total Calories _____ Carbs % ____ Protein % ____ Fat % ____

NOTES ON TODAY'S NUTRITION _____
_____
_____

How do you qualify your day? W ____ L ____

What went well? UPS

What did not go well? What is the plan to improve it tomorrow?

What did you learn about yourself today?

DAILY FITNESS TRACKER

Week Three – Day 4 – DATE: _____

Today's MSE GOAL – Upper – Lower – Core – HITT

Cardio

Activity	Minutes	Level/Speed Intensity	Heart Rate	Calories Burned	Notes

Strength

Exercise	SET 1 WT/REP	SET 2 WT/REP	SET 3 WT/REP	SET 4 WT/REP	Remarks

Stretching/Mobility

Activity/Move	REPS/TIME	Notes

ENDOMORPH @ WAR
LEVEL 1 – DAILY COMMITMENT

QUIT   COMPLIANT   OBSSESSED
WHY?

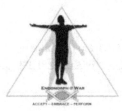

ENDOMORPH @ WAR
LEVEL ONE - DAILY REVIEW

DAILY RULES OF ENGAGEMENT

DATE_____

Today's Weight _____ BG (Tue/Fri)_____ BP _____

- ❏ Do something physical today 30+ minutes.
- ❏ Limit Carbs to less than 175 a day
- ❏ Don't drink your calories.
- ❏ Eat for Fuel, not for joy (change your relationship with food)
- ❏ Stay under 2,500 on workout days and U2K on non-workout days
- ❏ Kept the Fitness Schedule

Notes on Daily Battle;
_____
_____

FOOD INTAKE
Total Calories _____ Carbs % ____ Protein % ____ Fat % ____

NOTES ON TODAY'S NUTRITION
_____
_____
_____

How do you qualify your day? W ____ L ____

What went well? UPS

What did not go well? What is the plan to improve it tomorrow?

What did you learn about yourself today?

DAILY FITNESS TRACKER

Week Three – Day 5 – DATE: _____

Today's MSE GOAL – Upper – Lower – Core – HITT

Cardio

Activity	Minutes	Level/Speed Intensity	Heart Rate	Calories Burned	Notes

Strength

Exercise	SET 1 WT/REP	SET 2 WT/REP	SET 3 WT/REP	SET 4 WT/REP	Remarks

Stretching/Mobility

Activity/Move	REPS/TIME	Notes

ENDOMORPH @ WAR		
LEVEL 1 — DAILY COMMITMENT		
QUIT WHY?	COMPLIANT	OBSESSED

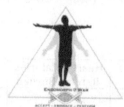

ENDOMORPH @ WAR
LEVEL ONE - DAILY REVIEW
DAILY RULES OF ENGAGEMENT

DATE_____

Today's Weight _____ BG (Tue/Fri) _____ BP _____

- ☐ Do something physical today 30+ minutes.
- ☐ Limit Carbs to less than 175 a day
- ☐ Don't drink your calories.
- ☐ Eat for Fuel, not for joy (change your relationship with food)
- ☐ Stay under 2,500 on workout days and U2K on non-workout days
- ☐ Kept the Fitness Schedule

Notes on Daily Battle:
_____
_____

FOOD INTAKE
Total Calories _____ Carbs % ____ Protein % ____ Fat % ____

NOTES ON TODAY'S NUTRITION
_____
_____
_____

How do you qualify your day? W ____ L ____

What went well? UPS

What did not go well? What is the plan to improve it tomorrow?

What did you learn about yourself today?

DAILY FITNESS TRACKER

Week Three – Day 6 – DATE: _____

Today's MSE GOAL – Upper – Lower – Core – HITT

Cardio

Activity	Minutes	Level/Speed Intensity	Heart Rate	Calories Burned	Notes

Strength

Exercise	SET 1 WT/REP	SET 2 WT/REP	SET 3 WT/REP	SET 4 WT/REP	Remarks

Stretching/Mobility

Activity/Move	REPS/TIME	Notes

| ENDOMORPH @ WAR |
| LEVEL 1 — DAILY COMMITMENT |

| QUIT WHY? | COMPLIANT | OBSSESSED |

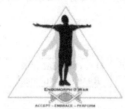

ENDOMORPH @ WAR
LEVEL ONE - DAILY REVIEW
DAILY RULES OF ENGAGEMENT

DATE_____

Today's Weight _____ BG (Tue/Fri) _____ BP _____

- ☐ Do something physical today 30+ minutes.
- ☐ Limit Carbs to less than 175 a day
- ☐ Don't drink your calories.
- ☐ Eat for Fuel, not for joy (change your relationship with food)
- ☐ Stay under 2,500 on workout days and U2K on non-workout days
- ☐ Kept the Fitness Schedule

Notes on Daily Battle;
_____
_____

FOOD INTAKE
Total Calories _____ Carbs % ____ Protein % ____ Fat % ____

NOTES ON TODAY'S NUTRITION
_____
_____
_____

How do you qualify your day? W ____ L ____

What went well? UPS

What did not go well? What is the plan to improve it tomorrow?

What did you learn about yourself today?

Week Three Notes

Week Four Matrix

SUN	MON	TUE	WED	THU	FRI	SAT

GOAL PROGRESS TRACKER

Goal	Date	Date	Date	Date	Date	Date

DAILY FITNESS TRACKER

Week Four – Day 1 – DATE: _____

Today's MSE GOAL – Upper – Lower – Core – HITT

Cardio

Activity	Minutes	Level/Speed Intensity	Heart Rate	Calories Burned	Notes

Strength

Exercise	SET 1 WT/REP	SET 2 WT/REP	SET 3 WT/REP	SET 4 WT/REP	Remarks

Stretching/Mobility

Activity/Move	REPS/TIME	Notes

ENDOMORPH @ WAR
LEVEL 1 — DAILY COMMITMENT

QUIT — COMPLIANT — OBSSESSED

WHY?

ENDOMORPH @ WAR
LEVEL ONE - DAILY REVIEW
DAILY RULES OF ENGAGEMENT

DATE_____

Today's Weight _____ BG (Tue/Fri) _____ BP _____

- ☐ Do something physical today 30+ minutes.
- ☐ Limit Carbs to less than 175 a day
- ☐ Don't drink your calories.
- ☐ Eat for Fuel, not for joy (change your relationship with food)
- ☐ Stay under 2,500 on workout days and U2K on non-workout days
- ☐ Kept the Fitness Schedule

Notes on Daily Battle;
_____
_____

FOOD INTAKE
Total Calories _____ Carbs % ____ Protein % ____ Fat % ____

NOTES ON TODAY'S NUTRITION
_____
_____
_____

How do you qualify your day? W ____ L ____

What went well? UPS

What did not go well? What is the plan to improve it tomorrow?

What did you learn about yourself today?

DAILY FITNESS TRACKER

Week Four – Day 2 – DATE: _____

Today's MSE GOAL – Upper – Lower – Core – HITT

Cardio

Activity	Minutes	Level/Speed Intensity	Heart Rate	Calories Burned	Notes

Strength

Exercise	SET 1 WT/REP	SET 2 WT/REP	SET 3 WT/REP	SET 4 WT/REP	Remarks

Stretching/Mobility

Activity/Move	REPS/TIME	Notes

ENDOMORPH @ WAR
LEVEL 1 — DAILY COMMITMENT

QUIT   COMPLIANT   OBSSESSED
WHY?

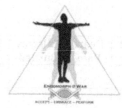

ENDOMORPH @ WAR
LEVEL ONE - DAILY REVIEW
DAILY RULES OF ENGAGEMENT

DATE_____

Today's Weight _____ BG (Tue/Fri) _____ BP _____

- ☐ Do something physical today 30+ minutes.
- ☐ Limit Carbs to less than 175 a day
- ☐ Don't drink your calories.
- ☐ Eat for Fuel, not for joy (change your relationship with food)
- ☐ Stay under 2,500 on workout days and U2K on non-workout days
- ☐ Kept the Fitness Schedule

Notes on Daily Battle:
_____
_____

FOOD INTAKE
Total Calories _____ Carbs % ____ Protein % ____ Fat % ____

NOTES ON TODAY'S NUTRITION
_____
_____
_____

How do you qualify your day? W ____ L ____

What went well? UPS

What did not go well? What is the plan to improve it tomorrow?

What did you learn about yourself today?

DAILY FITNESS TRACKER

Week Four – Day 3 – DATE: _____

Today's MSE GOAL – Upper – Lower – Core – HITT

Cardio

Activity	Minutes	Level/Speed Intensity	Heart Rate	Calories Burned	Notes

Strength

Exercise	SET 1 WT/REP	SET 2 WT/REP	SET 3 WT/REP	SET 4 WT/REP	Remarks

Stretching/Mobility

Activity/Move	REPS/TIME	Notes

ENDOMORPH @ WAR
LEVEL 1 — DAILY COMMITMENT

QUIT   COMPLIANT   OBSSESSED
WHY?

ENDOMORPH @ WAR
LEVEL ONE - DAILY REVIEW
DAILY RULES OF ENGAGEMENT

DATE_____

Today's Weight _____ BG (Tue/Fri) _____ BP _____

- ☐ Do something physical today 30+ minutes.
- ☐ Limit Carbs to less than 175 a day
- ☐ Don't drink your calories.
- ☐ Eat for Fuel, not for joy (change your relationship with food)
- ☐ Stay under 2,500 on workout days and U2K on non-workout days
- ☐ Kept the Fitness Schedule

Notes on Daily Battle:
_____
_____

FOOD INTAKE
Total Calories _____ Carbs % ____ Protein % ____ Fat % ____

NOTES ON TODAY'S NUTRITION
_____
_____
_____

How do you qualify your day? W ____ L ____

What went well? UPS

What did not go well? What is the plan to improve it tomorrow?

What did you learn about yourself today?

DAILY FITNESS TRACKER

Week Four – Day 4 – DATE: _____

Today's MSE GOAL – Upper – Lower – Core – HITT

Cardio

Activity	Minutes	Level/Speed Intensity	Heart Rate	Calories Burned	Notes

Strength

Exercise	SET 1 WT/REP	SET 2 WT/REP	SET 3 WT/REP	SET 4 WT/REP	Remarks

Stretching/Mobility

Activity/Move	REPS/TIME	Notes

ENDOMORPH @ WAR
LEVEL 1 – DAILY COMMITMENT

⇐──────────────────────────────────────⇒

QUIT   COMPLIANT   OBSSESSED
WHY?

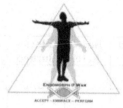

ENDOMORPH @ WAR
LEVEL ONE - DAILY REVIEW

DAILY RULES OF ENGAGEMENT

DATE_____

Today's Weight _____ BG (Tue/Fri) _____ BP _____

- ☐ Do something physical today 30+ minutes.
- ☐ Limit Carbs to less than 175 a day
- ☐ Don't drink your calories.
- ☐ Eat for Fuel, not for joy (change your relationship with food)
- ☐ Stay under 2,500 on workout days and U2K on non-workout days
- ☐ Kept the Fitness Schedule

Notes on Daily Battle;
_____
_____

FOOD INTAKE
Total Calories _____ Carbs % ____ Protein % ____ Fat % ____

NOTES ON TODAY'S NUTRITION
_____
_____
_____

How do you qualify your day? W ____ L ____

What went well? UPS

What did not go well? What is the plan to improve it tomorrow?

What did you learn about yourself today?

DAILY FITNESS TRACKER

Week Four – Day 5 – DATE: _____

Today's MSE GOAL – Upper – Lower – Core – HITT

Cardio

Activity	Minutes	Level/Speed Intensity	Heart Rate	Calories Burned	Notes

Strength

Exercise	SET 1 WT/REP	SET 2 WT/REP	SET 3 WT/REP	SET 4 WT/REP	Remarks

Stretching/Mobility

Activity/Move	REPS/TIME	Notes

ENDOMORPH @ WAR
LEVEL 1 – DAILY COMMITMENT

QUIT	COMPLIANT	OBSSESSED

WHY?

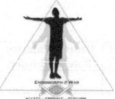

ENDOMORPH @ WAR
LEVEL ONE - DAILY REVIEW
DAILY RULES OF ENGAGEMENT

DATE_____

Today's Weight _____ BG (Tue/Fri)_____ BP _____

- ☐ Do something physical today 30+ minutes.
- ☐ Limit Carbs to less than 175 a day
- ☐ Don't drink your calories.
- ☐ Eat for Fuel, not for joy (change your relationship with food)
- ☐ Stay under 2,500 on workout days and U2K on non-workout days
- ☐ Kept the Fitness Schedule

Notes on Daily Battle;
_____
_____

FOOD INTAKE
Total Calories _____ Carbs % ____ Protein % ____ Fat % ____

NOTES ON TODAY'S NUTRITION
_____
_____
_____

How do you qualify your day? W ____ L ____

What went well? UPS

What did not go well? What is the plan to improve it tomorrow?

What did you learn about yourself today?

DAILY FITNESS TRACKER

Week Four – Day 6 – DATE: _____

Today's MSE GOAL – Upper – Lower – Core – HITT

Cardio

Activity	Minutes	Level/Speed Intensity	Heart Rate	Calories Burned	Notes

Strength

Exercise	SET 1 WT/REP	SET 2 WT/REP	SET 3 WT/REP	SET 4 WT/REP	Remarks

Stretching/Mobility

Activity/Move	REPS/TIME	Notes

ENDOMORPH @ WAR
LEVEL 1 — DAILY COMMITMENT

QUIT   COMPLIANT   OBSSESSED
WHY?

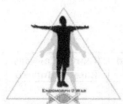

ENDOMORPH @ WAR
LEVEL ONE - DAILY REVIEW

DAILY RULES OF ENGAGEMENT

DATE _____

Today's Weight _____ BG (Tue/Fri) _____ BP _____

- ☐ Do something physical today 30+ minutes.
- ☐ Limit Carbs to less than 175 a day
- ☐ Don't drink your calories.
- ☐ Eat for Fuel, not for joy (change your relationship with food)
- ☐ Stay under 2,500 on workout days and U2K on non-workout days
- ☐ Kept the Fitness Schedule

Notes on Daily Battle:
_____
_____

FOOD INTAKE
Total Calories _____ Carbs % _____ Protein % _____ Fat % _____

NOTES ON TODAY'S NUTRITION
_____
_____
_____

How do you qualify your day? W _____ L _____

What went well? UPS

What did not go well? What is the plan to improve it tomorrow?

What did you learn about yourself today?

Week Four Notes

Week Five Matrix

SUN	MON	TUE	WED	THU	FRI	SAT

GOAL PROGRESS TRACKER

Goal	Date	Date	Date	Date	Date	Date

DAILY FITNESS TRACKER

Week Five – Day 1 – DATE: _____

Today's MSE GOAL – Upper – Lower – Core – HITT

Cardio

Activity	Minutes	Level/Speed Intensity	Heart Rate	Calories Burned	Notes

Strength

Exercise	SET 1 WT/REP	SET 2 WT/REP	SET 3 WT/REP	SET 4 WT/REP	Remarks

Stretching/Mobility

Activity/Move	REPS/TIME	Notes

ENDOMORPH @ WAR
LEVEL 1 — DAILY COMMITMENT

QUIT   COMPLIANT   OBSSESSED

WHY?

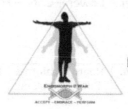

ENDOMORPH @ WAR
LEVEL ONE - DAILY REVIEW
DAILY RULES OF ENGAGEMENT

DATE_____

Today's Weight _____ BG (Tue/Fri) _____ BP _____

- ☐ Do something physical today 30+ minutes.
- ☐ Limit Carbs to less than 175 a day
- ☐ Don't drink your calories.
- ☐ Eat for Fuel, not for joy (change your relationship with food)
- ☐ Stay under 2,500 on workout days and U2K on non-workout days
- ☐ Kept the Fitness Schedule

Notes on Daily Battle;
_____
_____

FOOD INTAKE
Total Calories _____ Carbs % ____ Protein % ____ Fat % ____

NOTES ON TODAY'S NUTRITION
_____
_____
_____

How do you qualify your day? W ____ L ____

What went well? UPS

What did not go well? What is the plan to improve it tomorrow?

What did you learn about yourself today?

DAILY FITNESS TRACKER

Week Five – Day 2 – DATE: _____

Today's MSE GOAL – Upper – Lower – Core – HITT

Cardio

Activity	Minutes	Level/Speed Intensity	Heart Rate	Calories Burned	Notes

Strength

Exercise	SET 1 WT/REP	SET 2 WT/REP	SET 3 WT/REP	SET 4 WT/REP	Remarks

Stretching/Mobility

Activity/Move	REPS/TIME	Notes

| **ENDOMORPH @ WAR** |
| **LEVEL 1 – DAILY COMMITMENT** |

| QUIT | COMPLIANT | OBSSESSED |

WHY?

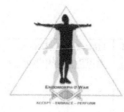

ENDOMORPH @ WAR
LEVEL ONE - DAILY REVIEW

DAILY RULES OF ENGAGEMENT

DATE_____

Today's Weight _____ BG (Tue/Fri)_____ BP _____

- ☐ Do something physical today 30+ minutes.
- ☐ Limit Carbs to less than 175 a day
- ☐ Don't drink your calories.
- ☐ Eat for Fuel, not for joy (change your relationship with food)
- ☐ Stay under 2,500 on workout days and U2K on non-workout days
- ☐ Kept the Fitness Schedule

Notes on Daily Battle;
_____
_____

FOOD INTAKE
Total Calories _____ Carbs % ____ Protein % ____ Fat % ____

NOTES ON TODAY'S NUTRITION
_____
_____
_____

How do you qualify your day? W ____ L ____

What went well? UPS

What did not go well? What is the plan to improve it tomorrow?

What did you learn about yourself today?

DAILY FITNESS TRACKER

Week Five – Day 3 – DATE: _____

Today's MSE GOAL – Upper – Lower – Core – HITT

Cardio

Activity	Minutes	Level/Speed Intensity	Heart Rate	Calories Burned	Notes

Strength

Exercise	SET 1 WT/REP	SET 2 WT/REP	SET 3 WT/REP	SET 4 WT/REP	Remarks

Stretching/Mobility

Activity/Move	REPS/TIME	Notes

ENDOMORPH @ WAR
LEVEL 1 — DAILY COMMITMENT

QUIT   COMPLIANT   OBSSESSED
WHY?

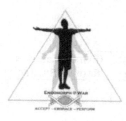

ENDOMORPH @ WAR
LEVEL ONE - DAILY REVIEW
DAILY RULES OF ENGAGEMENT

DATE_____

Today's Weight _____ BG (Tue/Fri)_____ BP _____

- ☐ Do something physical today 30+ minutes.
- ☐ Limit Carbs to less than 175 a day
- ☐ Don't drink your calories.
- ☐ Eat for Fuel, not for joy (change your relationship with food)
- ☐ Stay under 2,500 on workout days and U2K on non-workout days
- ☐ Kept the Fitness Schedule

Notes on Daily Battle:
_____
_____

FOOD INTAKE
Total Calories _____ Carbs % ____ Protein % ____ Fat % ____

NOTES ON TODAY'S NUTRITION
_____
_____
_____

How do you qualify your day? W ____ L ____

What went well? UPS

What did not go well? What is the plan to improve it tomorrow?

What did you learn about yourself today?

DAILY FITNESS TRACKER

Week Five – Day 4 – DATE: _____

Today's MSE GOAL – Upper – Lower – Core – HITT

Cardio

Activity	Minutes	Level/Speed Intensity	Heart Rate	Calories Burned	Notes

Strength

Exercise	SET 1 WT/REP	SET 2 WT/REP	SET 3 WT/REP	SET 4 WT/REP	Remarks

Stretching/Mobility

Activity/Move	REPS/TIME	Notes

ENDOMORPH @ WAR
LEVEL 1 — DAILY COMMITMENT

◄───►

QUIT   COMPLIANT   OBSSESSED
WHY?

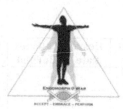

ENDOMORPH @ WAR
LEVEL ONE - DAILY REVIEW

DAILY RULES OF ENGAGEMENT

DATE_____

Today's Weight _____ BG (Tue/Fri) _____ BP _____

- ☐ Do something physical today 30+ minutes.
- ☐ Limit Carbs to less than 175 a day
- ☐ Don't drink your calories.
- ☐ Eat for Fuel, not for joy (change your relationship with food)
- ☐ Stay under 2,500 on workout days and U2K on non-workout days
- ☐ Kept the Fitness Schedule

Notes on Daily Battle:
_____
_____

FOOD INTAKE
Total Calories _____ Carbs % ____ Protein % ____ Fat % ____

NOTES ON TODAY'S NUTRITION
_____
_____
_____

How do you qualify your day? W ____ L ____

What went well? UPS

What did not go well? What is the plan to improve it tomorrow?

What did you learn about yourself today?

DAILY FITNESS TRACKER

Week Five – Day 5 – DATE: _____

Today's MSE GOAL – Upper – Lower – Core – HITT

Cardio

Activity	Minutes	Level/Speed Intensity	Heart Rate	Calories Burned	Notes

Strength

Exercise	SET 1 WT/REP	SET 2 WT/REP	SET 3 WT/REP	SET 4 WT/REP	Remarks

Stretching/Mobility

Activity/Move	REPS/TIME	Notes

ENDOMORPH @ WAR
LEVEL 1 — DAILY COMMITMENT

QUIT   COMPLIANT   OBSSESSED
WHY?

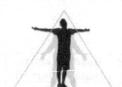

ENDOMORPH @ WAR
LEVEL ONE - DAILY REVIEW
DAILY RULES OF ENGAGEMENT

DATE_____

Today's Weight _____ BG (Tue/Fri) _____ BP _____

- ☐ Do something physical today 30+ minutes.
- ☐ Limit Carbs to less than 175 a day
- ☐ Don't drink your calories.
- ☐ Eat for Fuel, not for joy (change your relationship with food)
- ☐ Stay under 2,500 on workout days and U2K on non-workout days
- ☐ Kept the Fitness Schedule

Notes on Daily Battle:
_____
_____

FOOD INTAKE
Total Calories _____ Carbs % ____ Protein % ____ Fat % ____

NOTES ON TODAY'S NUTRITION
_____
_____
_____

How do you qualify your day? W ____ L ____

What went well? UPS

What did not go well? What is the plan to improve it tomorrow?

What did you learn about yourself today?

DAILY FITNESS TRACKER

Week Five – Day 6 – DATE: _____

Today's MSE GOAL – Upper – Lower – Core – HITT

Cardio

Activity	Minutes	Level/Speed Intensity	Heart Rate	Calories Burned	Notes

Strength

Exercise	SET 1 WT/REP	SET 2 WT/REP	SET 3 WT/REP	SET 4 WT/REP	Remarks

Stretching/Mobility

Activity/Move	REPS/TIME	Notes

ENDOMORPH @ WAR
LEVEL 1 — DAILY COMMITMENT

QUIT   COMPLIANT   OBSSESSED
WHY?

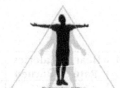

ENDOMORPH @ WAR
LEVEL ONE - DAILY REVIEW
DAILY RULES OF ENGAGEMENT

DATE_____

Today's Weight _____ BG (Tue/Fri) _____ BP _____

- ☐ Do something physical today 30+ minutes.
- ☐ Limit Carbs to less than 175 a day
- ☐ Don't drink your calories.
- ☐ Eat for Fuel, not for joy (change your relationship with food)
- ☐ Stay under 2,500 on workout days and U2K on non-workout days
- ☐ Kept the Fitness Schedule

Notes on Daily Battle;
_____
_____

FOOD INTAKE
Total Calories _____ Carbs % ____ Protein % ____ Fat % ____

NOTES ON TODAY'S NUTRITION
_____
_____
_____

How do you qualify your day? W ____ L ____

What went well? UPS

What did not go well? What is the plan to improve it tomorrow?

What did you learn about yourself today?

Week Five Notes

Week Six Matrix

SUN	MON	TUE	WED	THU	FRI	SAT

GOAL PROGRESS TRACKER

Goal	Date	Date	Date	Date	Date	Date

DAILY FITNESS TRACKER

Week Six – Day 1 – DATE: _____

Today's MSE GOAL – Upper – Lower – Core – HITT

Cardio

Activity	Minutes	Level/Speed Intensity	Heart Rate	Calories Burned	Notes

Strength

Exercise	SET 1 WT/REP	SET 2 WT/REP	SET 3 WT/REP	SET 4 WT/REP	Remarks

Stretching/Mobility

Activity/Move	REPS/TIME	Notes

```
ENDOMORPH @ WAR
LEVEL 1 — DAILY COMMITMENT
```

QUIT	COMPLIANT	OBSSESSED
WHY?		

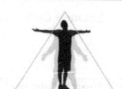

ENDOMORPH @ WAR
LEVEL ONE - DAILY REVIEW

DAILY RULES OF ENGAGEMENT

DATE_____

Today's Weight _____ BG (Tue/Fri)_____ BP _____

- ☐ Do something physical today 30+ minutes.
- ☐ Limit Carbs to less than 175 a day
- ☐ Don't drink your calories.
- ☐ Eat for Fuel, not for joy (change your relationship with food)
- ☐ Stay under 2,500 on workout days and U2K on non-workout days
- ☐ Kept the Fitness Schedule

Notes on Daily Battle:
_____
_____

FOOD INTAKE
Total Calories _____ Carbs % ____ Protein % ____ Fat % ____

NOTES ON TODAY'S NUTRITION
_____
_____
_____

How do you qualify your day? W ____ L ____

What went well? UPS

What did not go well? What is the plan to improve it tomorrow?

What did you learn about yourself today?

DAILY FITNESS TRACKER

Week Six – Day 2 – DATE: _____

Today's MSE GOAL – Upper – Lower – Core – HITT

Cardio

Activity	Minutes	Level/Speed Intensity	Heart Rate	Calories Burned	Notes

Strength

Exercise	SET 1 WT/REP	SET 2 WT/REP	SET 3 WT/REP	SET 4 WT/REP	Remarks

Stretching/Mobility

Activity/Move	REPS/TIME	Notes

ENDOMORPH @ WAR
LEVEL 1 – DAILY COMMITMENT

QUIT   COMPLIANT   OBSSESSED
WHY?

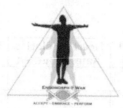

ENDOMORPH @ WAR
LEVEL ONE - DAILY REVIEW
DAILY RULES OF ENGAGEMENT

DATE_____

Today's Weight _____ BG (Tue/Fri)_____ BP _____

- ☐ Do something physical today 30+ minutes.
- ☐ Limit Carbs to less than 175 a day
- ☐ Don't drink your calories.
- ☐ Eat for Fuel, not for joy (change your relationship with food)
- ☐ Stay under 2,500 on workout days and U2K on non-workout days
- ☐ Kept the Fitness Schedule

Notes on Daily Battle;
_____
_____

FOOD INTAKE
Total Calories _____ Carbs % ____ Protein % ____ Fat % ____

NOTES ON TODAY'S NUTRITION
_____
_____
_____

How do you qualify your day? W ____ L ____

What went well? UPS

What did not go well? What is the plan to improve it tomorrow?

What did you learn about yourself today?

DAILY FITNESS TRACKER

Week Six – Day 3 – DATE: _____

Today's MSE GOAL – Upper – Lower – Core – HITT

Cardio

Activity	Minutes	Level/Speed Intensity	Heart Rate	Calories Burned	Notes

Strength

Exercise	SET 1 WT/REP	SET 2 WT/REP	SET 3 WT/REP	SET 4 WT/REP	Remarks

Stretching/Mobility

Activity/Move	REPS/TIME	Notes

ENDOMORPH @ WAR
LEVEL 1 — DAILY COMMITMENT

QUIT   COMPLIANT   OBSSESSED
WHY?

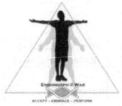

ENDOMORPH @ WAR
LEVEL ONE - DAILY REVIEW

DAILY RULES OF ENGAGEMENT

DATE_____

Today's Weight _____ BG (Tue/Fri)_____ BP _____

- ☐ Do something physical today 30+ minutes.
- ☐ Limit Carbs to less than 175 a day
- ☐ Don't drink your calories.
- ☐ Eat for Fuel, not for joy (change your relationship with food)
- ☐ Stay under 2,500 on workout days and U2K on non-workout days
- ☐ Kept the Fitness Schedule

Notes on Daily Battle;
_____
_____

FOOD INTAKE
Total Calories _____ Carbs % ____ Protein % ____ Fat % ____

NOTES ON TODAY'S NUTRITION
_____
_____
_____

How do you qualify your day? W ____ L ____

What went well? UPS

What did not go well? What is the plan to improve it tomorrow?

What did you learn about yourself today?

DAILY FITNESS TRACKER

Week Six – Day 4 – DATE: _____

Today's MSE GOAL – Upper – Lower – Core – HITT

Cardio

Activity	Minutes	Level/Speed Intensity	Heart Rate	Calories Burned	Notes

Strength

Exercise	SET 1 WT/REP	SET 2 WT/REP	SET 3 WT/REP	SET 4 WT/REP	Remarks

Stretching/Mobility

Activity/Move	REPS/TIME	Notes

ENDOMORPH @ WAR
LEVEL 1 — DAILY COMMITMENT

← QUIT   COMPLIANT   OBSSESSED →
WHY?

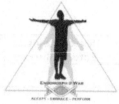

ENDOMORPH @ WAR
LEVEL ONE - DAILY REVIEW
DAILY RULES OF ENGAGEMENT

DATE_____

Today's Weight _____ BG (Tue/Fri) _____ BP _____

- ☐ Do something physical today 30+ minutes.
- ☐ Limit Carbs to less than 175 a day
- ☐ Don't drink your calories.
- ☐ Eat for Fuel, not for joy (change your relationship with food)
- ☐ Stay under 2,500 on workout days and U2K on non-workout days
- ☐ Kept the Fitness Schedule

Notes on Daily Battle:
_____
_____

FOOD INTAKE
Total Calories _____ Carbs % ____ Protein % ____ Fat % ____

NOTES ON TODAY'S NUTRITION
_____
_____
_____

How do you qualify your day? W ____ L ____

What went well? UPS

What did not go well? What is the plan to improve it tomorrow?

What did you learn about yourself today?

DAILY FITNESS TRACKER

Week Six – Day 5 – DATE: _____

Today's MSE GOAL – Upper – Lower – Core – HITT

Cardio

Activity	Minutes	Level/Speed Intensity	Heart Rate	Calories Burned	Notes

Strength

Exercise	SET 1 WT/REP	SET 2 WT/REP	SET 3 WT/REP	SET 4 WT/REP	Remarks

Stretching/Mobility

Activity/Move	REPS/TIME	Notes

ENDOMORPH @ WAR
LEVEL 1 – DAILY COMMITMENT

QUIT COMPLIANT OBSSESSED
WHY?

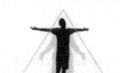

ENDOMORPH @ WAR
LEVEL ONE - DAILY REVIEW

DAILY RULES OF ENGAGEMENT

DATE_____

Today's Weight _____ BG (Tue/Fri) _____ BP _____

- ☐ Do something physical today 30+ minutes.
- ☐ Limit Carbs to less than 175 a day
- ☐ Don't drink your calories.
- ☐ Eat for Fuel, not for joy (change your relationship with food)
- ☐ Stay under 2,500 on workout days and U2K on non-workout days
- ☐ Kept the Fitness Schedule

Notes on Daily Battle;
_____
_____

FOOD INTAKE
Total Calories _____ Carbs % ___ Protein % ___ Fat % ___

NOTES ON TODAY'S NUTRITION
_____
_____
_____

How do you qualify your day? W ___ L ___

What went well? UPS

What did not go well? What is the plan to improve it tomorrow?

What did you learn about yourself today?

DAILY FITNESS TRACKER

Week Six – Day 6 – DATE: _____

Today's MSE GOAL – Upper – Lower – Core – HITT

Cardio

Activity	Minutes	Level/Speed Intensity	Heart Rate	Calories Burned	Notes

Strength

Exercise	SET 1 WT/REP	SET 2 WT/REP	SET 3 WT/REP	SET 4 WT/REP	Remarks

Stretching/Mobility

Activity/Move	REPS/TIME	Notes

ENDOMORPH @ WAR
LEVEL 1 – DAILY COMMITMENT

QUIT   COMPLIANT   OBSSESSED

WHY?

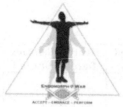

ENDOMORPH @ WAR
LEVEL ONE - DAILY REVIEW
DAILY RULES OF ENGAGEMENT

DATE_____

Today's Weight _____ BG (Tue/Fri) _____ BP _____

- ❏ Do something physical today 30+ minutes.
- ❏ Limit Carbs to less than 175 a day
- ❏ Don't drink your calories.
- ❏ Eat for Fuel, not for joy (change your relationship with food)
- ❏ Stay under 2,500 on workout days and U2K on non-workout days
- ❏ Kept the Fitness Schedule

Notes on Daily Battle:
_____
_____

FOOD INTAKE
Total Calories _____ Carbs % ____ Protein % ____ Fat % ____

NOTES ON TODAY'S NUTRITION
_____
_____
_____

How do you qualify your day? W ____ L ____

What went well? UPS

What did not go well? What is the plan to improve it tomorrow?

What did you learn about yourself today?

Week Six Notes

Week Seven Matrix

SUN	MON	TUE	WED	THU	FRI	SAT

GOAL PROGRESS TRACKER

Goal	Date	Date	Date	Date	Date	Date

DAILY FITNESS TRACKER

Week Seven – Day 1 – DATE: _____

Today's MSE GOAL – Upper – Lower – Core – HITT

Cardio

Activity	Minutes	Level/Speed Intensity	Heart Rate	Calories Burned	Notes

Strength

Exercise	SET 1 WT/REP	SET 2 WT/REP	SET 3 WT/REP	SET 4 WT/REP	Remarks

Stretching/Mobility

Activity/Move	REPS/TIME	Notes

ENDOMORPH @ WAR
LEVEL 1 — DAILY COMMITMENT

QUIT   COMPLIANT   OBSSESSED
WHY?

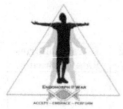

ENDOMORPH @ WAR
LEVEL ONE - DAILY REVIEW
DAILY RULES OF ENGAGEMENT

DATE_____

Today's Weight _____ BG (Tue/Fri)_____ BP _____

- ☐ Do something physical today 30+ minutes.
- ☐ Limit Carbs to less than 175 a day
- ☐ Don't drink your calories.
- ☐ Eat for Fuel, not for joy (change your relationship with food)
- ☐ Stay under 2,500 on workout days and U2K on non-workout days
- ☐ Kept the Fitness Schedule

Notes on Daily Battle;
_____
_____

FOOD INTAKE
Total Calories _____ Carbs % ____ Protein % ____ Fat % ____

NOTES ON TODAY'S NUTRITION
_____
_____
_____

How do you qualify your day? W ____ L ____

What went well? UPS

What did not go well? What is the plan to improve it tomorrow?

What did you learn about yourself today?

DAILY FITNESS TRACKER

Week Seven – Day 2 – DATE: _____

Today's MSE GOAL – Upper – Lower – Core – HITT

Cardio

Activity	Minutes	Level/Speed Intensity	Heart Rate	Calories Burned	Notes

Strength

Exercise	SET 1 WT/REP	SET 2 WT/REP	SET 3 WT/REP	SET 4 WT/REP	Remarks

Stretching/Mobility

Activity/Move	REPS/TIME	Notes

ENDOMORPH @ WAR
LEVEL 1 — DAILY COMMITMENT

| QUIT | COMPLIANT | OBSSESSED |

WHY?

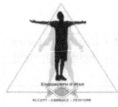

ENDOMORPH @ WAR
LEVEL ONE - DAILY REVIEW

DAILY RULES OF ENGAGEMENT

DATE_____

Today's Weight _____ BG (Tue/Fri) _____ BP _____

- ☐ Do something physical today 30+ minutes.
- ☐ Limit Carbs to less than 175 a day
- ☐ Don't drink your calories.
- ☐ Eat for Fuel, not for joy (change your relationship with food)
- ☐ Stay under 2,500 on workout days and U2K on non-workout days
- ☐ Kept the Fitness Schedule

Notes on Daily Battle;
_____
_____

FOOD INTAKE

Total Calories _____ Carbs % ____ Protein % ____ Fat % ____

NOTES ON TODAY'S NUTRITION
_____
_____
_____

How do you qualify your day? W ____ L ____

What went well? UPS

What did not go well? What is the plan to improve it tomorrow?

What did you learn about yourself today?

DAILY FITNESS TRACKER

Week Seven – Day 3 – DATE: _____

Today's MSE GOAL – Upper – Lower – Core – HITT

Cardio

Activity	Minutes	Level/Speed Intensity	Heart Rate	Calories Burned	Notes

Strength

Exercise	SET 1 WT/REP	SET 2 WT/REP	SET 3 WT/REP	SET 4 WT/REP	Remarks

Stretching/Mobility

Activity/Move	REPS/TIME	Notes

ENDOMORPH @ WAR
LEVEL 1 – DAILY COMMITMENT

| QUIT WHY? | COMPLIANT | OBSSESSED |

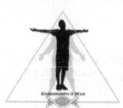

ENDOMORPH @ WAR
LEVEL ONE - DAILY REVIEW
DAILY RULES OF ENGAGEMENT

DATE_____

Today's Weight _____ BG (Tue/Fri) _____ BP _____

- ☐ Do something physical today 30+ minutes.
- ☐ Limit Carbs to less than 175 a day
- ☐ Don't drink your calories.
- ☐ Eat for Fuel, not for joy (change your relationship with food)
- ☐ Stay under 2,500 on workout days and U2K on non-workout days
- ☐ Kept the Fitness Schedule

Notes on Daily Battle:
_____
_____

FOOD INTAKE
Total Calories _____ Carbs % ____ Protein % ____ Fat % ____

NOTES ON TODAY'S NUTRITION
_____
_____
_____

How do you qualify your day? W ____ L ____

What went well? UPS

What did not go well? What is the plan to improve it tomorrow?

What did you learn about yourself today?

DAILY FITNESS TRACKER

Week Seven – Day 4 – DATE: _____

Today's MSE GOAL – Upper – Lower – Core – HITT

Cardio

Activity	Minutes	Level/Speed Intensity	Heart Rate	Calories Burned	Notes

Strength

Exercise	SET 1 WT/REP	SET 2 WT/REP	SET 3 WT/REP	SET 4 WT/REP	Remarks

Stretching/Mobility

Activity/Move	REPS/TIME	Notes

ENDOMORPH @ WAR
LEVEL 1 – DAILY COMMITMENT

QUIT	COMPLIANT	OBSSESSED
WHY?		

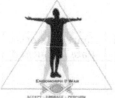

ENDOMORPH @ WAR
LEVEL ONE - DAILY REVIEW
DAILY RULES OF ENGAGEMENT
DATE_____

Today's Weight _____ BG (Tue/Fri) _____ BP _____

- ❏ Do something physical today 30+ minutes.
- ❏ Limit Carbs to less than 175 a day
- ❏ Don't drink your calories.
- ❏ Eat for Fuel, not for joy (change your relationship with food)
- ❏ Stay under 2,500 on workout days and U2K on non-workout days
- ❏ Kept the Fitness Schedule

Notes on Daily Battle:
_____
_____

FOOD INTAKE
Total Calories _____ Carbs % ____ Protein % ____ Fat % ____

NOTES ON TODAY'S NUTRITION
_____
_____
_____

How do you qualify your day? W _____ L _____

What went well? UPS

What did not go well? What is the plan to improve it tomorrow?

What did you learn about yourself today?

DAILY FITNESS TRACKER

Week Seven – Day 5 – DATE: _____

Today's MSE GOAL – Upper – Lower – Core – HITT

Cardio

Activity	Minutes	Level/Speed Intensity	Heart Rate	Calories Burned	Notes

Strength

Exercise	SET 1 WT/REP	SET 2 WT/REP	SET 3 WT/REP	SET 4 WT/REP	Remarks

Stretching/Mobility

Activity/Move	REPS/TIME	Notes

ENDOMORPH @ WAR
LEVEL 1 – DAILY COMMITMENT

QUIT	COMPLIANT	OBSSESSED
WHY?		

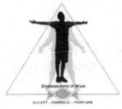

ENDOMORPH @ WAR
LEVEL ONE - DAILY REVIEW
DAILY RULES OF ENGAGEMENT

DATE_____

Today's Weight _____ BG (Tue/Fri)_____ BP _____

- ☐ Do something physical today 30+ minutes.
- ☐ Limit Carbs to less than 175 a day
- ☐ Don't drink your calories.
- ☐ Eat for Fuel, not for joy (change your relationship with food)
- ☐ Stay under 2,500 on workout days and U2K on non-workout days
- ☐ Kept the Fitness Schedule

Notes on Daily Battle;
_____
_____

FOOD INTAKE
Total Calories _____ Carbs % ____ Protein % ____ Fat % ____

NOTES ON TODAY'S NUTRITION
_____
_____
_____

How do you qualify your day? W ____ L ____

What went well? UPS

What did not go well? What is the plan to improve it tomorrow?

What did you learn about yourself today?

DAILY FITNESS TRACKER

Week Seven – Day 6 – DATE: _____

Today's MSE GOAL – Upper – Lower – Core – HITT

Cardio

Activity	Minutes	Level/Speed Intensity	Heart Rate	Calories Burned	Notes

Strength

Exercise	SET 1 WT/REP	SET 2 WT/REP	SET 3 WT/REP	SET 4 WT/REP	Remarks

Stretching/Mobility

Activity/Move	REPS/TIME	Notes

ENDOMORPH @ WAR
LEVEL 1 — DAILY COMMITMENT

QUIT   COMPLIANT   OBSSESSED
WHY?

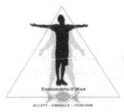

ENDOMORPH @ WAR
LEVEL ONE - DAILY REVIEW
DAILY RULES OF ENGAGEMENT

DATE_____

Today's Weight _____ BG (Tue/Fri)_____ BP _____

- ☐ Do something physical today 30+ minutes.
- ☐ Limit Carbs to less than 175 a day
- ☐ Don't drink your calories.
- ☐ Eat for Fuel, not for joy (change your relationship with food)
- ☐ Stay under 2,500 on workout days and U2K on non-workout days
- ☐ Kept the Fitness Schedule

Notes on Daily Battle;
_____
_____

FOOD INTAKE
Total Calories _____ Carbs % ____ Protein % ____ Fat % ____

NOTES ON TODAY'S NUTRITION
_____
_____
_____

How do you qualify your day? W ____ L ____

What went well? UPS

What did not go well? What is the plan to improve it tomorrow?

What did you learn about yourself today?

Week Seven Notes

Week Eight Matrix

SUN	MON	TUE	WED	THU	FRI	SAT

GOAL PROGRESS TRACKER

Goal	Date	Date	Date	Date	Date	Date

DAILY FITNESS TRACKER

Week Eight – Day 1 – DATE: _____

Today's MSE GOAL – Upper – Lower – Core – HITT

Cardio

Activity	Minutes	Level/Speed Intensity	Heart Rate	Calories Burned	Notes

Strength

Exercise	SET 1 WT/REP	SET 2 WT/REP	SET 3 WT/REP	SET 4 WT/REP	Remarks

Stretching/Mobility

Activity/Move	REPS/TIME	Notes

ENDOMORPH @ WAR
LEVEL 1 – DAILY COMMITMENT

QUIT — COMPLIANT — OBSSESSED
WHY?

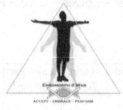

ENDOMORPH @ WAR
LEVEL ONE - DAILY REVIEW
DAILY RULES OF ENGAGEMENT

DATE_____

Today's Weight _____ BG (Tue/Fri)_____ BP _____

- ☐ Do something physical today 30+ minutes.
- ☐ Limit Carbs to less than 175 a day
- ☐ Don't drink your calories.
- ☐ Eat for Fuel, not for joy (change your relationship with food)
- ☐ Stay under 2,500 on workout days and U2K on non-workout days
- ☐ Kept the Fitness Schedule

Notes on Daily Battle;
_____
_____

FOOD INTAKE
Total Calories _____ Carbs % ____ Protein % ____ Fat % ____

NOTES ON TODAY'S NUTRITION
_____
_____
_____

How do you qualify your day? W____ L____

What went well? UPS

What did not go well? What is the plan to improve it tomorrow?

What did you learn about yourself today?

DAILY FITNESS TRACKER

Week Eight – Day 2 – DATE: _____

Today's MSE GOAL – Upper – Lower – Core – HITT

Cardio

Activity	Minutes	Level/Speed Intensity	Heart Rate	Calories Burned	Notes

Strength

Exercise	SET 1 WT/REP	SET 2 WT/REP	SET 3 WT/REP	SET 4 WT/REP	Remarks

Stretching/Mobility

Activity/Move	REPS/TIME	Notes

| ENDOMORPH @ WAR |
| LEVEL 1 – DAILY COMMITMENT |

| QUIT | COMPLIANT | OBSSESSED |
| WHY? | | |

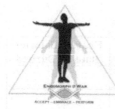

ENDOMORPH @ WAR
LEVEL ONE - DAILY REVIEW
DAILY RULES OF ENGAGEMENT

DATE_____

Today's Weight _____ BG (Tue/Fri)_____ BP _____

- ❏ Do something physical today 30+ minutes.
- ❏ Limit Carbs to less than 175 a day
- ❏ Don't drink your calories.
- ❏ Eat for Fuel, not for joy (change your relationship with food)
- ❏ Stay under 2,500 on workout days and U2K on non-workout days
- ❏ Kept the Fitness Schedule

Notes on Daily Battle;
_____
_____

FOOD INTAKE
Total Calories _____ Carbs % ____ Protein % ____ Fat % ____

NOTES ON TODAY'S NUTRITION
_____
_____
_____

How do you qualify your day? W ____ L ____

What went well? UPS

What did not go well? What is the plan to improve it tomorrow?

What did you learn about yourself today?

DAILY FITNESS TRACKER

Week Eight – Day 3 – DATE: _____

Today's MSE GOAL – Upper – Lower – Core – HITT

Cardio

Activity	Minutes	Level/Speed Intensity	Heart Rate	Calories Burned	Notes

Strength

Exercise	SET 1 WT/REP	SET 2 WT/REP	SET 3 WT/REP	SET 4 WT/REP	Remarks

Stretching/Mobility

Activity/Move	REPS/TIME	Notes

ENDOMORPH @ WAR
LEVEL 1 — DAILY COMMITMENT

QUIT   COMPLIANT   OBSSESSED
WHY?

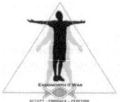

ENDOMORPH @ WAR
LEVEL ONE - DAILY REVIEW
DAILY RULES OF ENGAGEMENT

DATE_____

Today's Weight _____ BG (Tue/Fri) _____ BP _____

- ☐ Do something physical today 30+ minutes.
- ☐ Limit Carbs to less than 175 a day
- ☐ Don't drink your calories.
- ☐ Eat for Fuel, not for joy (change your relationship with food)
- ☐ Stay under 2,500 on workout days and U2K on non-workout days
- ☐ Kept the Fitness Schedule

Notes on Daily Battle;
_____
_____

FOOD INTAKE
Total Calories _____ Carbs % ____ Protein % ____ Fat % ____

NOTES ON TODAY'S NUTRITION
_____
_____
_____

How do you qualify your day? W ____ L ____

What went well? UPS

What did not go well? What is the plan to improve it tomorrow?

What did you learn about yourself today?

DAILY FITNESS TRACKER

Week Eight – Day 4 – DATE: _____

Today's MSE GOAL – Upper – Lower – Core – HITT

Cardio

Activity	Minutes	Level/Speed Intensity	Heart Rate	Calories Burned	Notes

Strength

Exercise	SET 1 WT/REP	SET 2 WT/REP	SET 3 WT/REP	SET 4 WT/REP	Remarks

Stretching/Mobility

Activity/Move	REPS/TIME	Notes

ENDOMORPH @ WAR
LEVEL 1 – DAILY COMMITMENT

QUIT   COMPLIANT   OBSSESSED
WHY?

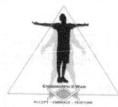

ENDOMORPH @ WAR
LEVEL ONE - DAILY REVIEW

DAILY RULES OF ENGAGEMENT

DATE_____

Today's Weight _____ BG (Tue/Fri) _____ BP _____

- ❑ Do something physical today 30+ minutes.
- ❑ Limit Carbs to less than 175 a day
- ❑ Don't drink your calories.
- ❑ Eat for Fuel, not for joy (change your relationship with food)
- ❑ Stay under 2,500 on workout days and U2K on non-workout days
- ❑ Kept the Fitness Schedule

Notes on Daily Battle;
_____
_____

FOOD INTAKE
Total Calories _____ Carbs % ____ Protein % ____ Fat % ____

NOTES ON TODAY'S NUTRITION
_____
_____
_____

How do you qualify your day? W ____ L ____

What went well? UPS

What did not go well? What is the plan to improve it tomorrow?

What did you learn about yourself today?

DAILY FITNESS TRACKER

Week Eight – Day 5 – DATE: _____

Today's MSE GOAL – Upper – Lower – Core – HITT

Cardio

Activity	Minutes	Level/Speed Intensity	Heart Rate	Calories Burned	Notes

Strength

Exercise	SET 1 WT/REP	SET 2 WT/REP	SET 3 WT/REP	SET 4 WT/REP	Remarks

Stretching/Mobility

Activity/Move	REPS/TIME	Notes

ENDOMORPH @ WAR
LEVEL 1 — DAILY COMMITMENT

QUIT   COMPLIANT   OBSSESSED
WHY?

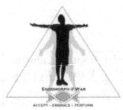

ENDOMORPH @ WAR
LEVEL ONE - DAILY REVIEW
DAILY RULES OF ENGAGEMENT

DATE_____

Today's Weight _____ BG (Tue/Fri) _____ BP _____

- ☐ Do something physical today 30+ minutes.
- ☐ Limit Carbs to less than 175 a day
- ☐ Don't drink your calories.
- ☐ Eat for Fuel, not for joy (change your relationship with food)
- ☐ Stay under 2,500 on workout days and U2K on non-workout days
- ☐ Kept the Fitness Schedule

Notes on Daily Battle;
_____
_____

FOOD INTAKE
Total Calories _____ Carbs % ____ Protein % ____ Fat % ____

NOTES ON TODAY'S NUTRITION
_____
_____
_____

How do you qualify your day? W ____ L ____

What went well? UPS

What did not go well? What is the plan to improve it tomorrow?

What did you learn about yourself today?

DAILY FITNESS TRACKER

Week Eight – Day 6 – DATE: _____

Today's MSE GOAL – Upper – Lower – Core – HITT

Cardio

Activity	Minutes	Level/Speed Intensity	Heart Rate	Calories Burned	Notes

Strength

Exercise	SET 1 WT/REP	SET 2 WT/REP	SET 3 WT/REP	SET 4 WT/REP	Remarks

Stretching/Mobility

Activity/Move	REPS/TIME	Notes

ENDOMORPH @ WAR
LEVEL 1 – DAILY COMMITMENT

QUIT	COMPLIANT	OBSSESSED
WHY?		

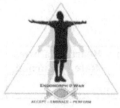

ENDOMORPH @ WAR
LEVEL ONE - DAILY REVIEW
DAILY RULES OF ENGAGEMENT

DATE_____

Today's Weight _____ BG (Tue/Fri)_____ BP _____

- ☐ Do something physical today 30+ minutes.
- ☐ Limit Carbs to less than 175 a day
- ☐ Don't drink your calories.
- ☐ Eat for Fuel, not for joy (change your relationship with food)
- ☐ Stay under 2,500 on workout days and U2K on non-workout days
- ☐ Kept the Fitness Schedule

Notes on Daily Battle;
_____
_____

FOOD INTAKE
Total Calories _____ Carbs % ____ Protein % ____ Fat % ____

NOTES ON TODAY'S NUTRITION
_____
_____
_____

How do you qualify your day? W ____ L ____

What went well? UPS

What did not go well? What is the plan to improve it tomorrow?

What did you learn about yourself today?

Week Eight Notes

Week Nine Matrix

SUN	MON	TUE	WED	THU	FRI	SAT

GOAL PROGRESS TRACKER

Goal	Date	Date	Date	Date	Date	Date

DAILY FITNESS TRACKER

Week Nine – Day 1 – DATE: _____

Today's MSE GOAL – Upper – Lower – Core – HITT

Cardio

Activity	Minutes	Level/Speed Intensity	Heart Rate	Calories Burned	Notes

Strength

Exercise	SET 1 WT/REP	SET 2 WT/REP	SET 3 WT/REP	SET 4 WT/REP	Remarks

Stretching/Mobility

Activity/Move	REPS/TIME	Notes

ENDOMORPH @ WAR
LEVEL 1 – DAILY COMMITMENT

QUIT	COMPLIANT	OBSSESSED
WHY?		

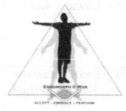

ENDOMORPH @ WAR
LEVEL ONE - DAILY REVIEW

DAILY RULES OF ENGAGEMENT

DATE_____

Today's Weight _____ BG (Tue/Fri) _____ BP _____

- ☐ Do something physical today 30+ minutes.
- ☐ Limit Carbs to less than 175 a day
- ☐ Don't drink your calories.
- ☐ Eat for Fuel, not for joy (change your relationship with food)
- ☐ Stay under 2,500 on workout days and U2K on non-workout days
- ☐ Kept the Fitness Schedule

Notes on Daily Battle;
_____
_____

FOOD INTAKE
Total Calories _____ Carbs % ____ Protein % ____ Fat % ____

NOTES ON TODAY'S NUTRITION
_____
_____
_____

How do you qualify your day? W ____ L ____

What went well? UPS

What did not go well? What is the plan to improve it tomorrow?

What did you learn about yourself today?

DAILY FITNESS TRACKER

Week Nine – Day 2 – DATE: _____

Today's MSE GOAL – Upper – Lower – Core – HITT

Cardio

Activity	Minutes	Level/Speed Intensity	Heart Rate	Calories Burned	Notes

Strength

Exercise	SET 1 WT/REP	SET 2 WT/REP	SET 3 WT/REP	SET 4 WT/REP	Remarks

Stretching/Mobility

Activity/Move	REPS/TIME	Notes

ENDOMORPH @ WAR
LEVEL 1 – DAILY COMMITMENT

QUIT   COMPLIANT   OBSSESSED
WHY?

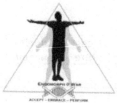

ENDOMORPH @ WAR
LEVEL ONE - DAILY REVIEW
DAILY RULES OF ENGAGEMENT

DATE_____

Today's Weight _____ BG (Tue/Fri)_____ BP _____

- ☐ Do something physical today 30+ minutes.
- ☐ Limit Carbs to less than 175 a day
- ☐ Don't drink your calories.
- ☐ Eat for Fuel, not for joy (change your relationship with food)
- ☐ Stay under 2,500 on workout days and U2K on non-workout days
- ☐ Kept the Fitness Schedule

Notes on Daily Battle;
_____
_____

FOOD INTAKE
Total Calories _____ Carbs % _____ Protein % _____ Fat % _____

NOTES ON TODAY'S NUTRITION
_____
_____
_____

How do you qualify your day? W _____ L _____

What went well? UPS

What did not go well? What is the plan to improve it tomorrow?

What did you learn about yourself today?

DAILY FITNESS TRACKER

Week Nine – Day 3 – DATE: _____

Today's MSE GOAL – Upper – Lower – Core – HITT

Cardio

Activity	Minutes	Level/Speed Intensity	Heart Rate	Calories Burned	Notes

Strength

Exercise	SET 1 WT/REP	SET 2 WT/REP	SET 3 WT/REP	SET 4 WT/REP	Remarks

Stretching/Mobility

Activity/Move	REPS/TIME	Notes

ENDOMORPH @ WAR
LEVEL 1 – DAILY COMMITMENT

| QUIT | COMPLIANT | OBSSESSED |

WHY?

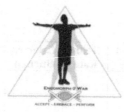

ENDOMORPH @ WAR
LEVEL ONE - DAILY REVIEW
DAILY RULES OF ENGAGEMENT

DATE_____

Today's Weight _____ BG (Tue/Fri) _____ BP _____

- ☐ Do something physical today 30+ minutes.
- ☐ Limit Carbs to less than 175 a day
- ☐ Don't drink your calories.
- ☐ Eat for Fuel, not for joy (change your relationship with food)
- ☐ Stay under 2,500 on workout days and U2K on non-workout days
- ☐ Kept the Fitness Schedule

Notes on Daily Battle;
_____
_____

FOOD INTAKE
Total Calories _____ Carbs % ____ Protein % ____ Fat % ____

NOTES ON TODAY'S NUTRITION
_____
_____
_____

How do you qualify your day? W ____ L ____

What went well? UPS

What did not go well? What is the plan to improve it tomorrow?

What did you learn about yourself today?

DAILY FITNESS TRACKER

Week Nine – Day 4 – DATE: _____

Today's MSE GOAL – Upper – Lower – Core – HITT

Cardio

Activity	Minutes	Level/Speed Intensity	Heart Rate	Calories Burned	Notes

Strength

Exercise	SET 1 WT/REP	SET 2 WT/REP	SET 3 WT/REP	SET 4 WT/REP	Remarks

Stretching/Mobility

Activity/Move	REPS/TIME	Notes

ENDOMORPH @ WAR
LEVEL 1 – DAILY COMMITMENT

QUIT   COMPLIANT   OBSSESSED
WHY?

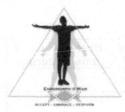

ENDOMORPH @ WAR
LEVEL ONE - DAILY REVIEW

DAILY RULES OF ENGAGEMENT

DATE_____

Today's Weight _____ BG (Tue/Fri)_____ BP _____

- ☐ Do something physical today 30+ minutes.
- ☐ Limit Carbs to less than 175 a day
- ☐ Don't drink your calories.
- ☐ Eat for Fuel, not for joy (change your relationship with food)
- ☐ Stay under 2,500 on workout days and U2K on non-workout days
- ☐ Kept the Fitness Schedule

Notes on Daily Battle;
_____
_____

FOOD INTAKE
Total Calories _____ Carbs % ____ Protein % ____ Fat % ____

NOTES ON TODAY'S NUTRITION
_____
_____
_____

How do you qualify your day? W ____ L ____

What went well? UPS

What did not go well? What is the plan to improve it tomorrow?

What did you learn about yourself today?

DAILY FITNESS TRACKER

Week Nine – Day 5 – DATE: _____

Today's MSE GOAL – Upper – Lower – Core – HITT

Cardio

Activity	Minutes	Level/Speed Intensity	Heart Rate	Calories Burned	Notes

Strength

Exercise	SET 1 WT/REP	SET 2 WT/REP	SET 3 WT/REP	SET 4 WT/REP	Remarks

Stretching/Mobility

Activity/Move	REPS/TIME	Notes

ENDOMORPH @ WAR
LEVEL 1 – DAILY COMMITMENT

QUIT   COMPLIANT   OBSSESSED

WHY?

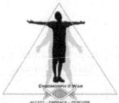

ENDOMORPH @ WAR
LEVEL ONE - DAILY REVIEW

DAILY RULES OF ENGAGEMENT

DATE_____

Today's Weight _____ BG (Tue/Fri)_____ BP _____

- ☐ Do something physical today 30+ minutes.
- ☐ Limit Carbs to less than 175 a day
- ☐ Don't drink your calories.
- ☐ Eat for Fuel, not for joy (change your relationship with food)
- ☐ Stay under 2,500 on workout days and U2K on non-workout days
- ☐ Kept the Fitness Schedule

Notes on Daily Battle;
_____
_____

FOOD INTAKE
Total Calories _____ Carbs % ____ Protein % ____ Fat % ____

NOTES ON TODAY'S NUTRITION
_____
_____
_____

How do you qualify your day? W ____ L ____

What went well? UPS

What did not go well? What is the plan to improve it tomorrow?

What did you learn about yourself today?

DAILY FITNESS TRACKER

Week Nine – Day 6 – DATE: _____

Today's MSE GOAL – Upper – Lower – Core – HITT

Cardio

Activity	Minutes	Level/Speed Intensity	Heart Rate	Calories Burned	Notes

Strength

Exercise	SET 1 WT/REP	SET 2 WT/REP	SET 3 WT/REP	SET 4 WT/REP	Remarks

Stretching/Mobility

Activity/Move	REPS/TIME	Notes

ENDOMORPH @ WAR
LEVEL 1 — DAILY COMMITMENT

QUIT   COMPLIANT   OBSSESSED

WHY?

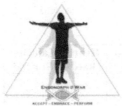

ENDOMORPH @ WAR
LEVEL ONE - DAILY REVIEW
DAILY RULES OF ENGAGEMENT

DATE_____

Today's Weight _____ BG (Tue/Fri)_____ BP _____

- ☐ Do something physical today 30+ minutes.
- ☐ Limit Carbs to less than 175 a day
- ☐ Don't drink your calories.
- ☐ Eat for Fuel, not for joy (change your relationship with food)
- ☐ Stay under 2,500 on workout days and U2K on non-workout days
- ☐ Kept the Fitness Schedule

Notes on Daily Battle;
_____
_____

FOOD INTAKE

Total Calories _____ Carbs % ____ Protein % ____ Fat % ____

NOTES ON TODAY'S NUTRITION
_____
_____
_____

How do you qualify your day? W ____ L ____

What went well? UPS

What did not go well? What is the plan to improve it tomorrow?

What did you learn about yourself today?

Week Nine Notes

Week Ten Matrix

SUN	MON	TUE	WED	THU	FRI	SAT

GOAL PROGRESS TRACKER

Goal	Date	Date	Date	Date	Date	Date

DAILY FITNESS TRACKER

Week Ten – Day 1 – DATE: _____

Today's MSE GOAL – Upper – Lower – Core – HITT

Cardio

Activity	Minutes	Level/Speed Intensity	Heart Rate	Calories Burned	Notes

Strength

Exercise	SET 1 WT/REP	SET 2 WT/REP	SET 3 WT/REP	SET 4 WT/REP	Remarks

Stretching/Mobility

Activity/Move	REPS/TIME	Notes

ENDOMORPH @ WAR
LEVEL 1 – DAILY COMMITMENT

QUIT   COMPLIANT   OBSSESSED
WHY?

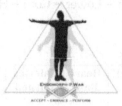

ENDOMORPH @ WAR
LEVEL ONE - DAILY REVIEW

DAILY RULES OF ENGAGEMENT

DATE_____

Today's Weight _____ BG (Tue/Fri) _____ BP _____

- ☐ Do something physical today 30+ minutes.
- ☐ Limit Carbs to less than 175 a day
- ☐ Don't drink your calories.
- ☐ Eat for Fuel, not for joy (change your relationship with food)
- ☐ Stay under 2,500 on workout days and U2K on non-workout days
- ☐ Kept the Fitness Schedule

Notes on Daily Battle;
_____
_____

FOOD INTAKE
Total Calories _____ Carbs % ____ Protein % ____ Fat % ____

NOTES ON TODAY'S NUTRITION
_____
_____
_____

How do you qualify your day? W ____ L ____

What went well? UPS

What did not go well? What is the plan to improve it tomorrow?

What did you learn about yourself today?

DAILY FITNESS TRACKER

Week Ten – Day 2 – DATE: _____

Today's MSE GOAL – Upper – Lower – Core – HITT

Cardio

Activity	Minutes	Level/Speed Intensity	Heart Rate	Calories Burned	Notes

Strength

Exercise	SET 1 WT/REP	SET 2 WT/REP	SET 3 WT/REP	SET 4 WT/REP	Remarks

Stretching/Mobility

Activity/Move	REPS/TIME	Notes

ENDOMORPH @ WAR
LEVEL 1 — DAILY COMMITMENT

QUIT	COMPLIANT	OBSSESSED
WHY?		

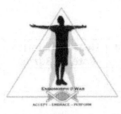

ENDOMORPH @ WAR
LEVEL ONE - DAILY REVIEW
DAILY RULES OF ENGAGEMENT

DATE_____

Today's Weight _____ BG (Tue/Fri) _____ BP _____

- ☐ Do something physical today 30+ minutes.
- ☐ Limit Carbs to less than 175 a day
- ☐ Don't drink your calories.
- ☐ Eat for Fuel, not for joy (change your relationship with food)
- ☐ Stay under 2,500 on workout days and U2K on non-workout days
- ☐ Kept the Fitness Schedule

Notes on Daily Battle;
_____
_____

FOOD INTAKE
Total Calories _____ Carbs % ____ Protein % ____ Fat % ____

NOTES ON TODAY'S NUTRITION
_____
_____
_____

How do you qualify your day? W ____ L ____

What went well? UPS

What did not go well? What is the plan to improve it tomorrow?

What did you learn about yourself today?

DAILY FITNESS TRACKER

Week Ten – Day 3 – DATE: _____

Today's MSE GOAL – Upper – Lower – Core – HITT

Cardio

Activity	Minutes	Level/Speed Intensity	Heart Rate	Calories Burned	Notes

Strength

Exercise	SET 1 WT/REP	SET 2 WT/REP	SET 3 WT/REP	SET 4 WT/REP	Remarks

Stretching/Mobility

Activity/Move	REPS/TIME	Notes

ENDOMORPH @ WAR
LEVEL 1 — DAILY COMMITMENT

QUIT WHY?   COMPLIANT   OBSSESSED

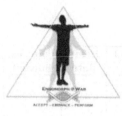

ENDOMORPH @ WAR
LEVEL ONE - DAILY REVIEW
DAILY RULES OF ENGAGEMENT

DATE_____

Today's Weight _____ BG (Tue/Fri)_____ BP _____

- ☐ Do something physical today 30+ minutes.
- ☐ Limit Carbs to less than 175 a day
- ☐ Don't drink your calories.
- ☐ Eat for Fuel, not for joy (change your relationship with food)
- ☐ Stay under 2,500 on workout days and U2K on non-workout days
- ☐ Kept the Fitness Schedule

Notes on Daily Battle;
_____
_____

FOOD INTAKE
Total Calories _____ Carbs % ____ Protein % ____ Fat % ____

NOTES ON TODAY'S NUTRITION
_____
_____
_____

How do you qualify your day? W ____ L ____

What went well? UPS

What did not go well? What is the plan to improve it tomorrow?

What did you learn about yourself today?

DAILY FITNESS TRACKER

Week Ten – Day 4 – DATE: _____

Today's MSE GOAL – Upper – Lower – Core – HITT

Cardio

Activity	Minutes	Level/Speed Intensity	Heart Rate	Calories Burned	Notes

Strength

Exercise	SET 1 WT/REP	SET 2 WT/REP	SET 3 WT/REP	SET 4 WT/REP	Remarks

Stretching/Mobility

Activity/Move	REPS/TIME	Notes

ENDOMORPH @ WAR
LEVEL 1 – DAILY COMMITMENT

QUIT　　　　　　　　　　COMPLIANT　　　　　　　　　　OBSSESSED
WHY?

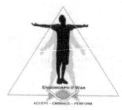

ENDOMORPH @ WAR
LEVEL ONE - DAILY REVIEW

DAILY RULES OF ENGAGEMENT

DATE_____

Today's Weight _____ BG (Tue/Fri) _____ BP _____

- ☐ Do something physical today 30+ minutes.
- ☐ Limit Carbs to less than 175 a day
- ☐ Don't drink your calories.
- ☐ Eat for Fuel, not for joy (change your relationship with food)
- ☐ Stay under 2,500 on workout days and U2K on non-workout days
- ☐ Kept the Fitness Schedule

Notes on Daily Battle;
_____
_____

FOOD INTAKE
Total Calories _____ Carbs % ____ Protein % ____ Fat % ____

NOTES ON TODAY'S NUTRITION
_____
_____
_____

How do you qualify your day? W ____ L ____

What went well? UPS

What did not go well? What is the plan to improve it tomorrow?

What did you learn about yourself today?

DAILY FITNESS TRACKER

Week Ten – Day 5 – DATE: _____

Today's MSE GOAL – Upper – Lower – Core – HITT

Cardio

Activity	Minutes	Level/Speed Intensity	Heart Rate	Calories Burned	Notes

Strength

Exercise	SET 1 WT/REP	SET 2 WT/REP	SET 3 WT/REP	SET 4 WT/REP	Remarks

Stretching/Mobility

Activity/Move	REPS/TIME	Notes

ENDOMORPH @ WAR
LEVEL 1 — DAILY COMMITMENT

QUIT	COMPLIANT	OBSSESSED
WHY?		

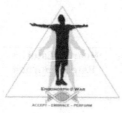

ENDOMORPH @ WAR
LEVEL ONE - DAILY REVIEW

DAILY RULES OF ENGAGEMENT

DATE_____

Today's Weight _____ BG (Tue/Fri)_____ BP _____

- ☐ Do something physical today 30+ minutes.
- ☐ Limit Carbs to less than 175 a day
- ☐ Don't drink your calories.
- ☐ Eat for Fuel, not for joy (change your relationship with food)
- ☐ Stay under 2,500 on workout days and U2K on non-workout days
- ☐ Kept the Fitness Schedule

Notes on Daily Battle:
_____
_____

FOOD INTAKE
Total Calories _____ Carbs % ____ Protein % ____ Fat % ____

NOTES ON TODAY'S NUTRITION
_____
_____
_____

How do you qualify your day? W ____ L ____

What went well? UPS

What did not go well? What is the plan to improve it tomorrow?

What did you learn about yourself today?

DAILY FITNESS TRACKER

Week Ten – Day 6 – DATE: _____

Today's MSE GOAL – Upper – Lower – Core – HITT

Cardio

Activity	Minutes	Level/Speed Intensity	Heart Rate	Calories Burned	Notes

Strength

Exercise	SET 1 WT/REP	SET 2 WT/REP	SET 3 WT/REP	SET 4 WT/REP	Remarks

Stretching/Mobility

Activity/Move	REPS/TIME	Notes

ENDOMORPH @ WAR
LEVEL 1 — DAILY COMMITMENT

QUIT   COMPLIANT   OBSSESSED

WHY?

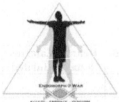

ENDOMORPH @ WAR
LEVEL ONE - DAILY REVIEW

DAILY RULES OF ENGAGEMENT

DATE_____

Today's Weight _____ BG (Tue/Fri) _____ BP _____

- ☐ Do something physical today 30+ minutes.
- ☐ Limit Carbs to less than 175 a day
- ☐ Don't drink your calories.
- ☐ Eat for Fuel, not for joy (change your relationship with food)
- ☐ Stay under 2,500 on workout days and U2K on non-workout days
- ☐ Kept the Fitness Schedule

Notes on Daily Battle;
_____
_____

FOOD INTAKE
Total Calories _____ Carbs % ____ Protein % ____ Fat % ____

NOTES ON TODAY'S NUTRITION
_____
_____
_____

How do you qualify your day? W ____ L ____

What went well? UPS

What did not go well? What is the plan to improve it tomorrow?

What did you learn about yourself today?

Week Ten Notes

Week 11 Matrix

SUN	MON	TUE	WED	THU	FRI	SAT

GOAL PROGRESS TRACKER

Goal	Date	Date	Date	Date	Date	Date

DAILY FITNESS TRACKER

Week 11 – Day 1 – DATE: _____

Today's MSE GOAL – Upper – Lower – Core – HITT

Cardio

Activity	Minutes	Level/Speed Intensity	Heart Rate	Calories Burned	Notes

Strength

Exercise	SET 1 WT/REP	SET 2 WT/REP	SET 3 WT/REP	SET 4 WT/REP	Remarks

Stretching/Mobility

Activity/Move	REPS/TIME	Notes

ENDOMORPH @ WAR
LEVEL 1 – DAILY COMMITMENT

QUIT	COMPLIANT	OBSSESSED
WHY?		

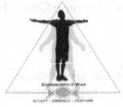

ENDOMORPH @ WAR
LEVEL ONE - DAILY REVIEW

DAILY RULES OF ENGAGEMENT

DATE_____

Today's Weight _____ BG (Tue/Fri)_____ BP _____

- ☐ Do something physical today 30+ minutes.
- ☐ Limit Carbs to less than 175 a day
- ☐ Don't drink your calories.
- ☐ Eat for Fuel, not for joy (change your relationship with food)
- ☐ Stay under 2,500 on workout days and U2K on non-workout days
- ☐ Kept the Fitness Schedule

Notes on Daily Battle:
_____
_____

FOOD INTAKE
Total Calories _____ Carbs % ____ Protein % ____ Fat % ____

NOTES ON TODAY'S NUTRITION
_____
_____
_____

How do you qualify your day? W ____ L ____

What went well? UPS

What did not go well? What is the plan to improve it tomorrow?

What did you learn about yourself today?

DAILY FITNESS TRACKER

Week 11 – Day 2 – DATE: _____

Today's MSE GOAL – Upper – Lower – Core – HITT

Cardio

Activity	Minutes	Level/Speed Intensity	Heart Rate	Calories Burned	Notes

Strength

Exercise	SET 1 WT/REP	SET 2 WT/REP	SET 3 WT/REP	SET 4 WT/REP	Remarks

Stretching/Mobility

Activity/Move	REPS/TIME	Notes

ENDOMORPH @ WAR
LEVEL 1 – DAILY COMMITMENT

QUIT — WHY?   COMPLIANT   OBSSESSED

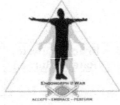

ENDOMORPH @ WAR
LEVEL ONE - DAILY REVIEW
DAILY RULES OF ENGAGEMENT

DATE_____

Today's Weight _____ BG (Tue/Fri) _____ BP _____

- ☐ Do something physical today 30+ minutes.
- ☐ Limit Carbs to less than 175 a day
- ☐ Don't drink your calories.
- ☐ Eat for Fuel, not for joy (change your relationship with food)
- ☐ Stay under 2,500 on workout days and U2K on non-workout days
- ☐ Kept the Fitness Schedule

Notes on Daily Battle;
_____
_____

FOOD INTAKE
Total Calories _____ Carbs % ____ Protein % ____ Fat % ____

NOTES ON TODAY'S NUTRITION
_____
_____
_____

How do you qualify your day? W ____ L ____

What went well? UPS

What did not go well? What is the plan to improve it tomorrow?

What did you learn about yourself today?

DAILY FITNESS TRACKER

Week 11 – Day 3 – DATE: _____

Today's MSE GOAL – Upper – Lower – Core – HITT

Cardio

Activity	Minutes	Level/Speed Intensity	Heart Rate	Calories Burned	Notes

Strength

Exercise	SET 1 WT/REP	SET 2 WT/REP	SET 3 WT/REP	SET 4 WT/REP	Remarks

Stretching/Mobility

Activity/Move	REPS/TIME	Notes

ENDOMORPH @ WAR
LEVEL 1 – DAILY COMMITMENT

QUIT　　　　　　　　　COMPLIANT　　　　　　　　　OBSSESSED
WHY?

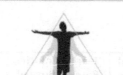

ENDOMORPH @ WAR
LEVEL ONE - DAILY REVIEW
DAILY RULES OF ENGAGEMENT

DATE_____

Today's Weight _____ BG (Tue/Fri)_____ BP _____

- ☐ Do something physical today 30+ minutes.
- ☐ Limit Carbs to less than 175 a day
- ☐ Don't drink your calories.
- ☐ Eat for Fuel, not for joy (change your relationship with food)
- ☐ Stay under 2,500 on workout days and U2K on non-workout days
- ☐ Kept the Fitness Schedule

Notes on Daily Battle;
_____
_____

FOOD INTAKE
Total Calories _____ Carbs % ____ Protein % ____ Fat % ____

NOTES ON TODAY'S NUTRITION
_____
_____
_____

How do you qualify your day? W ____ L ____

What went well? UPS

What did not go well? What is the plan to improve it tomorrow?

What did you learn about yourself today?

DAILY FITNESS TRACKER

Week 11 – Day 4 – DATE: _____

Today's MSE GOAL – Upper – Lower – Core – HITT

Cardio

Activity	Minutes	Level/Speed Intensity	Heart Rate	Calories Burned	Notes

Strength

Exercise	SET 1 WT/REP	SET 2 WT/REP	SET 3 WT/REP	SET 4 WT/REP	Remarks

Stretching/Mobility

Activity/Move	REPS/TIME	Notes

ENDOMORPH @ WAR
LEVEL 1 – DAILY COMMITMENT

| QUIT | COMPLIANT | OBSSESSED |
| WHY? | | |

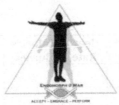

ENDOMORPH @ WAR
LEVEL ONE - DAILY REVIEW

DAILY RULES OF ENGAGEMENT

DATE_____

Today's Weight _____ BG (Tue/Fri)_____ BP _____

- ☐ Do something physical today 30+ minutes.
- ☐ Limit Carbs to less than 175 a day
- ☐ Don't drink your calories.
- ☐ Eat for Fuel, not for joy (change your relationship with food)
- ☐ Stay under 2,500 on workout days and U2K on non-workout days
- ☐ Kept the Fitness Schedule

Notes on Daily Battle;
_____
_____

FOOD INTAKE
Total Calories _____ Carbs % ____ Protein % ____ Fat % ____

NOTES ON TODAY'S NUTRITION
_____
_____
_____

How do you qualify your day? W ____ L ____

What went well? UPS

What did not go well? What is the plan to improve it tomorrow?

What did you learn about yourself today?

DAILY FITNESS TRACKER

Week 11 – Day 5 – DATE: _____

Today's MSE GOAL – Upper – Lower – Core – HITT

Cardio

Activity	Minutes	Level/Speed Intensity	Heart Rate	Calories Burned	Notes

Strength

Exercise	SET 1 WT/REP	SET 2 WT/REP	SET 3 WT/REP	SET 4 WT/REP	Remarks

Stretching/Mobility

Activity/Move	REPS/TIME	Notes

Endomorph @ War
Level 1 – Daily Commitment

QUIT   COMPLIANT   OBSSESSED
WHY?

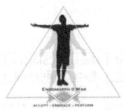

Endomorph @ War
Level One - Daily Review
Daily Rules of Engagement

DATE_____

Today's Weight _____ BG (Tue/Fri)_____ BP _____

- ☐ Do something physical today 30+ minutes.
- ☐ Limit Carbs to less than 175 a day
- ☐ Don't drink your calories.
- ☐ Eat for Fuel, not for joy (change your relationship with food)
- ☐ Stay under 2,500 on workout days and U2K on non-workout days
- ☐ Kept the Fitness Schedule

Notes on Daily Battle:
_____
_____

FOOD INTAKE
Total Calories _____ Carbs % ____ Protein % ____ Fat % ____

NOTES ON TODAY'S NUTRITION
_____
_____
_____

How do you qualify your day? W ____ L ____

What went well? UPS

What did not go well? What is the plan to improve it tomorrow?

What did you learn about yourself today?

DAILY FITNESS TRACKER

Week 11 – Day 6 – DATE: _____

Today's MSE GOAL – Upper – Lower – Core – HITT

Cardio

Activity	Minutes	Level/Speed Intensity	Heart Rate	Calories Burned	Notes

Strength

Exercise	SET 1 WT/REP	SET 2 WT/REP	SET 3 WT/REP	SET 4 WT/REP	Remarks

Stretching/Mobility

Activity/Move	REPS/TIME	Notes

ENDOMORPH @ WAR
LEVEL 1 – DAILY COMMITMENT

QUIT   COMPLIANT   OBSSESSED
WHY?

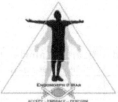

ENDOMORPH @ WAR
LEVEL ONE - DAILY REVIEW
DAILY RULES OF ENGAGEMENT

DATE_____

Today's Weight _____ BG (Tue/Fri) _____ BP _____

- ☐ Do something physical today 30+ minutes.
- ☐ Limit Carbs to less than 175 a day
- ☐ Don't drink your calories.
- ☐ Eat for Fuel, not for joy (change your relationship with food)
- ☐ Stay under 2,500 on workout days and U2K on non-workout days
- ☐ Kept the Fitness Schedule

Notes on Daily Battle:
_____
_____

FOOD INTAKE
Total Calories _____ Carbs % ____ Protein % ____ Fat % ____

NOTES ON TODAY'S NUTRITION
_____
_____
_____

How do you qualify your day? W ____ L ____

What went well? UPS

What did not go well? What is the plan to improve it tomorrow?

What did you learn about yourself today?

Week 11 Notes

Week 12 Matrix

SUN	MON	TUE	WED	THU	FRI	SAT

GOAL PROGRESS TRACKER

Goal	Date	Date	Date	Date	Date	Date

DAILY FITNESS TRACKER

Week 12 – Day 1 – DATE: _____

Today's MSE GOAL – Upper – Lower – Core – HITT

Cardio

Activity	Minutes	Level/Speed Intensity	Heart Rate	Calories Burned	Notes

Strength

Exercise	SET 1 WT/REP	SET 2 WT/REP	SET 3 WT/REP	SET 4 WT/REP	Remarks

Stretching/Mobility

Activity/Move	REPS/TIME	Notes

| ENDOMORPH @ WAR |
| LEVEL 1 – DAILY COMMITMENT |

| QUIT | COMPLIANT | OBSESSED |
| WHY? | | |

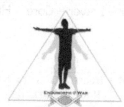

ENDOMORPH @ WAR
LEVEL ONE - DAILY REVIEW
DAILY RULES OF ENGAGEMENT
DATE_____

Today's Weight _____ BG (Tue/Fri) _____ BP _____

- ☐ Do something physical today 30+ minutes.
- ☐ Limit Carbs to less than 175 a day
- ☐ Don't drink your calories.
- ☐ Eat for Fuel, not for joy (change your relationship with food)
- ☐ Stay under 2,500 on workout days and U2K on non-workout days
- ☐ Kept the Fitness Schedule

Notes on Daily Battle;
_____
_____

FOOD INTAKE
Total Calories _____ Carbs % ____ Protein % ____ Fat % ____

NOTES ON TODAY'S NUTRITION
_____
_____
_____

How do you qualify your day? W ____ L ____

What went well? UPS

What did not go well? What is the plan to improve it tomorrow?

What did you learn about yourself today?

DAILY FITNESS TRACKER

Week 12 – Day 2 – DATE: _____

Today's MSE GOAL – Upper – Lower – Core – HITT

Cardio

Activity	Minutes	Level/Speed Intensity	Heart Rate	Calories Burned	Notes

Strength

Exercise	SET 1 WT/REP	SET 2 WT/REP	SET 3 WT/REP	SET 4 WT/REP	Remarks

Stretching/Mobility

Activity/Move	REPS/TIME	Notes

Endomorph @ War
Level 1 – Daily Commitment

QUIT — COMPLIANT — OBSSESSED
WHY?

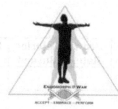

Endomorph @ War
Level One - Daily Review
Daily Rules of Engagement

DATE_____

Today's Weight _____ BG (Tue/Fri)_____ BP _____

- ☐ Do something physical today 30+ minutes.
- ☐ Limit Carbs to less than 175 a day
- ☐ Don't drink your calories.
- ☐ Eat for Fuel, not for joy (change your relationship with food)
- ☐ Stay under 2,500 on workout days and U2K on non-workout days
- ☐ Kept the Fitness Schedule

Notes on Daily Battle;
_____
_____

FOOD INTAKE
Total Calories _____ Carbs % _____ Protein % _____ Fat % _____

NOTES ON TODAY'S NUTRITION
_____
_____
_____

How do you qualify your day? W _____ L _____

What went well? UPS

What did not go well? What is the plan to improve it tomorrow?

What did you learn about yourself today?

DAILY FITNESS TRACKER

Week 12 – Day 3 – DATE: _____

Today's MSE GOAL – Upper – Lower – Core – HITT

Cardio

Activity	Minutes	Level/Speed Intensity	Heart Rate	Calories Burned	Notes

Strength

Exercise	SET 1 WT/REP	SET 2 WT/REP	SET 3 WT/REP	SET 4 WT/REP	Remarks

Stretching/Mobility

Activity/Move	REPS/TIME	Notes

ENDOMORPH @ WAR
LEVEL 1 – DAILY COMMITMENT

QUIT   COMPLIANT   OBSSESSED
WHY?

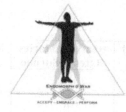

ENDOMORPH @ WAR
LEVEL ONE - DAILY REVIEW

DAILY RULES OF ENGAGEMENT

DATE_____

Today's Weight _____ BG (Tue/Fri) _____ BP _____

- ☐ Do something physical today 30+ minutes.
- ☐ Limit Carbs to less than 175 a day
- ☐ Don't drink your calories.
- ☐ Eat for Fuel, not for joy (change your relationship with food)
- ☐ Stay under 2,500 on workout days and U2K on non-workout days
- ☐ Kept the Fitness Schedule

Notes on Daily Battle:
_____
_____

FOOD INTAKE
Total Calories _____ Carbs % ____ Protein % ____ Fat % ____

NOTES ON TODAY'S NUTRITION
_____
_____
_____

How do you qualify your day? W ____ L ____

What went well? UPS

What did not go well? What is the plan to improve it tomorrow?

What did you learn about yourself today?

DAILY FITNESS TRACKER

Week 12 – Day 4 – DATE: _____

Today's MSE GOAL – Upper – Lower – Core – HITT

Cardio

Activity	Minutes	Level/Speed Intensity	Heart Rate	Calories Burned	Notes

Strength

Exercise	SET 1 WT/REP	SET 2 WT/REP	SET 3 WT/REP	SET 4 WT/REP	Remarks

Stretching/Mobility

Activity/Move	REPS/TIME	Notes

ENDOMORPH @ WAR
LEVEL 1 — DAILY COMMITMENT

QUIT　　　　　　　　　　COMPLIANT　　　　　　　　　　OBSSESSED
WHY?

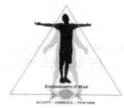

ENDOMORPH @ WAR
LEVEL ONE - DAILY REVIEW

DAILY RULES OF ENGAGEMENT

DATE_____

Today's Weight _____ BG (Tue/Fri)_____ BP _____

- ☐ Do something physical today 30+ minutes.
- ☐ Limit Carbs to less than 175 a day
- ☐ Don't drink your calories.
- ☐ Eat for Fuel, not for joy (change your relationship with food)
- ☐ Stay under 2,500 on workout days and U2K on non-workout days
- ☐ Kept the Fitness Schedule

Notes on Daily Battle;
_____
_____

FOOD INTAKE
Total Calories _____ Carbs % ____ Protein % ____ Fat % ____

NOTES ON TODAY'S NUTRITION
_____
_____
_____

How do you qualify your day? W ____ L ____

What went well? UPS

What did not go well? What is the plan to improve it tomorrow?

What did you learn about yourself today?

DAILY FITNESS TRACKER

Week 12 – Day 5 – DATE: _____

Today's MSE GOAL – Upper – Lower – Core – HITT

Cardio

Activity	Minutes	Level/Speed Intensity	Heart Rate	Calories Burned	Notes

Strength

Exercise	SET 1 WT/REP	SET 2 WT/REP	SET 3 WT/REP	SET 4 WT/REP	Remarks

Stretching/Mobility

Activity/Move	REPS/TIME	Notes

ENDOMORPH @ WAR
LEVEL 1 – DAILY COMMITMENT

QUIT   COMPLIANT   OBSSESSED

WHY?

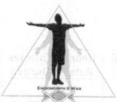

ENDOMORPH @ WAR
LEVEL ONE - DAILY REVIEW
DAILY RULES OF ENGAGEMENT

DATE_____

Today's Weight _____ BG (Tue/Fri) _____ BP _____

- ☐ Do something physical today 30+ minutes.
- ☐ Limit Carbs to less than 175 a day
- ☐ Don't drink your calories.
- ☐ Eat for Fuel, not for joy (change your relationship with food)
- ☐ Stay under 2,500 on workout days and U2K on non-workout days
- ☐ Kept the Fitness Schedule

Notes on Daily Battle;
_____
_____

FOOD INTAKE
Total Calories _____ Carbs % ____ Protein % ____ Fat % ____

NOTES ON TODAY'S NUTRITION
_____
_____
_____

How do you qualify your day? W ____ L ____

What went well? UPS

What did not go well? What is the plan to improve it tomorrow?

What did you learn about yourself today?

DAILY FITNESS TRACKER

Week 12 – Day 6 – DATE: _____

Today's MSE GOAL – Upper – Lower – Core – HITT

Cardio

Activity	Minutes	Level/Speed Intensity	Heart Rate	Calories Burned	Notes

Strength

Exercise	SET 1 WT/REP	SET 2 WT/REP	SET 3 WT/REP	SET 4 WT/REP	Remarks

Stretching/Mobility

Activity/Move	REPS/TIME	Notes

ENDOMORPH @ WAR
LEVEL 1 — DAILY COMMITMENT

◄───►

QUIT   COMPLIANT   OBSSESSED
WHY?

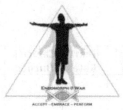

ENDOMORPH @ WAR
LEVEL ONE - DAILY REVIEW
DAILY RULES OF ENGAGEMENT

DATE_____

Today's Weight _____ BG (Tue/Fri)_____ BP _____

- ☐ Do something physical today 30+ minutes.
- ☐ Limit Carbs to less than 175 a day
- ☐ Don't drink your calories.
- ☐ Eat for Fuel, not for joy (change your relationship with food)
- ☐ Stay under 2,500 on workout days and U2K on non-workout days
- ☐ Kept the Fitness Schedule

Notes on Daily Battle:
_____
_____

FOOD INTAKE
Total Calories _____ Carbs % _____ Protein % _____ Fat % _____

NOTES ON TODAY'S NUTRITION
_____
_____
_____

How do you qualify your day? W _____ L _____

What went well? UPS

What did not go well? What is the plan to improve it tomorrow?

What did you learn about yourself today?

Week 12 Notes

About the Author

Dr. Morales-Negron attended the University of Puerto Rico where he completed a degree in physical education and received a 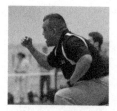 commission as an officer in the U.S. Army in 1990. He completed the U.S. Army Master Fitness Trainer course in 1993 and has helped thousands of soldiers in the development of personal fitness programs. Throughout his career, he has received certifications through the American Council of Sports Medicine (ACSM), American Council of Exercise (ACE), and Spinning among others. In 1998, he received a Masters in Kinesiology from the University of Georgia and became an instructor of physical education at the U.S. Military Academy at West Point. During his first tour at West Point, he instructed cadets in personal fitness, wellness, and unit fitness program development among other courses for three years. After leaving the academy, he was responsible for sports and fitness programs for Army Soldiers in South Korea and trained soldiers in Fort Bliss, Texas to lead the new Army Physical Readiness program in 2002.

In 2004, Dr Morales was selected to become an Academy Professor of Physical Education at West Point and became the first Hispanic in the history of West Point to be selected for this position. In 2005, he attended Florida State University to complete his doctorate in sport and exercise psychology. In 2008, after the completion of his requirements at FSU, he reported to the Department of Physical Education. As an Academy Professor, Dr Morales was responsible for the department's administrative duties, competitive clubs' administration, coaching the West Point Judo team, and served as course director for personal fitness, combatives instructor certification, basic Judo instruction, and nutrition for performance. In 2010, Dr Morales completed all the requirements to become a certified performance enhancement consultant through the Association for Applied Sport Psychology (AASP) and currently works with athletes in mental conditioning as well as individuals that need to set a path to achieve higher levels of performance, fitness, and wellness. In 2013, he received West Point's Brigadier General Anderson Award for Excellence in Teaching and in 2014 he received the Coach Mike Krizenski's Teaching Character through Sports Award.

In 2014, Dr. Morales retired from the U.S. Army after 26 years of wearing the military uniform. Since his retirement, DrM has been working with professional athletes providing guidance, direction, and mentorship for their performance journey.

Made in the USA
Middletown, DE
22 October 2024